AIDS
MYTHS, FACTS & ETHICS

AIDS
*M*YTHS, *F*ACTS & *E*THICS

ELIZABETH PRIOR JONSON

PERGAMON PRESS
SYDNEY • OXFORD • NEW YORK
BEIJING • FRANKFURT • SÃO PAULO • TOKYO • TORONTO

AUSTRALIA	Pergamon Press (Australia) Pty Ltd, 19a Boundary Street, Rushcutters Bay, NSW 2011, Australia
UK	Pergamon Press plc, Headington Hill Hall, Oxford OX3 OBW, England
USA	Pergamon Press, Inc., Maxwell House, Fairview Park, Elmsford, New York 10523, USA
PEOPLE'S REPUBLIC OF CHINA	Pergamon Press, Room 4037, Qianmen Hotel, Beijing, People's Republic of China
FEDERAL REPUBLIC OF GERMANY	Pergamon Press GmbH, Hammerweg 6, D-6242 Kronberg, Federal Republic of Germany
BRAZIL	Pergamon Editora Ltda, Rua Eca de Queiros, 346, CEP 04011, Paraiso, São Paulo, Brazil
JAPAN	Pergamon Press, 8th Floor, Matsuoka Central Building, 1-7-1 Nishishinjuku, Shinjuku-ku, Tokyo 160, Japan
CANADA	Pergamon Press Canada Ltd, Suite 271, 253 College Street, Toronto, Ontario M5T 1R5, Canada

First published 1988

Copyright ©Elizabeth Prior Jonson, 1988

Cover design by Hand Graphics

Typeset by Post Typesetters, Brisbane, Australia
Printed in Singapore by Singapore National Printers Ltd

National Library of Australia
Cataloguing in Publication data:

Prior Jonson, Elizabeth, 1952–
  AIDS: myths, facts and ethics.

  Includes bibliographies.
  ISBN 0 08 034434 8.

  1. AIDS (Disease) — Moral and ethical aspects.
  2. AIDS (Disease) — Law and legislation.
  3. AIDS (Disease) — Social aspects. I. Title.

362.1'969792

All rights reserved. No part of this publication may be reproduced, stored in a retrieval system or transmitted in any form or by any means, electronic, electrostatic, magnetic tape, mechanical, photocopying, recording or otherwise, without permission in writing from Pergamon Press (Australia) Pty. Ltd.

RA
644
.A25
P74
1988
c.1

CONTENTS

Acknowledgements	vi
Terms	vi
Introduction	vii
1 The Medical Facts	1
2 Ethics	12
3 AIDS, Ethics and Sex	30
4 From Ethics to Discriminatory Policies	45
5 What Is the Law For?	64
6 AIDS and the Criminal Law	77
7 Paternalism	96
8 Homosex and Heterosex	111
9 Prisons, Drugs and Kids	126
10 The Provision of Health Care	140
11 AIDS and You	155

Acknowledgements

Chapter 4 of this book, 'From Ethics to Discriminatory Policies', is co-authored with Robert Pargetter.

I would like to thank David Armstrong, Geoffrey Blainey, Peter Boxall, Jane Diplock, Peter Jonson, Robert Pargetter, Philip Pettit and Judy Thomson for their comments on, and criticisms of, versions of this work.

Terms

AIDS	Acquired Immune Deficiency Syndrome — the most serious form of HIV infection, which leads to death
ARC	AIDS Related Complex — a less serious form of HIV infection, which is not fatal
Antibody positive	Someone who has been tested and found to have HIV antibodies in his or her blood, but who may display no symptoms of HIV infection, is antibody positive. Such people *may transmit the virus to others.*
ceteris paribus	other things being equal
HIV	Human Immunodeficiency Virus
prima facie	at first glance

INTRODUCTION

AIDS has sometimes been referred to as a 'modern' or 'gay' plague, a 1980s version of the Black Death. Between 1347 and 1350 the bubonic plague swept through Europe. It is estimated that within those three years a third of the population — some 80 million people — were wiped out. In some cities 80 per cent of the population perished. People did not understand that the disease was carried by fleas living on rats. It seemed to them that any contact with a plague victim would result in further contagion and death. Physicians refused to attend patients, and the dead were left unburied. Husbands abandoned their sick wives, and parents their infected children. For AIDS to approach the scale of that plague it would have to kill one hundred million Europeans before 1990. Even the most pessimistic estimates fall far short of that.

Nevertheless, there have been many tragedies caused by AIDS. In 1985 three-year-old Eve Van Grafhorst became an overnight *cause célèbre* when she was excluded from a Gosford day care centre after it became known that she was infected with the AIDS virus. The Health Department later decided that she could return to the centre since she did not pose any substantial threat to the health of the other children, and that is when the trouble really started. The parents of the other children were simply not prepared to accept any risk, no matter how small. As one parent said: 'The majority of parents don't want to send their children to the centre if Eve is there, and the view of the majority is what democracy is based on, isn't it?'

More recently there has been the case involving Police Constable Andrew Dixon. Constable Dixon was splashed with blood while accompanying a road accident victim to hospital in an ambulance. Later he learnt that this man had AIDS. Constable Dixon became severely depressed believing himself to be infected and later shot himself. Experts estimate the probability that Dixon actually was infected as virtually non-existent.

Vocal reaction to AIDS has not been confined to those who perceive themselves or their families to be at immediate risk of HIV infection. Dr Jerry Falwell, president of the Moral Majority in the USA, has claimed that AIDS is divine retribution against homosexuals for breaking the laws of God and nature. Falwell has called for the closure of America's public bath houses which, in his view, are there only to provide a venue for promiscuous homosexual sex, and therefore should not be allowed.

In a similar vein, Dr Vernon Mark, neurosurgeon and professor at Harvard Medical School, has suggested that irresponsible AIDS carriers be quarantined on Penikese Island off Cape Cod, an island which, until 1922, was used as a leper colony. William F. Buckley, a luminary of the American right, has argued that 'everyone detected with AIDS should be tattooed on the upper forearm, to protect common needle users, and in the buttocks to prevent the victimisation of other homosexuals'.

Falwell's claim that AIDS is divine retribution upon homosexuals deserves little attention. After all, the 'innocent' wives of bisexual men may become infected even while being totally faithful to their husbands. And there are also 'innocent' children and babies who have become infected as the result of blood tranfusions, or because they were unlucky enough to have drug addicted mothers. But Falwell has raised other issues which must be treated more seriously. He argues that governments have failed to close bath houses and, more importantly, the US government has not taken action to prevent homosexuals from donating blood because of pressure exerted by the gay political lobby. Falwell correctly points out that the polio epidemic of the 1950s brought about the closure of public swimming pools, because these were seen to be venues for spreading the polio virus. Since AIDS is every bit as serious as polio, measures which may contribute significantly to halting its spread should be given suitable consideration.

Closer to home, Professor David Pennington, former head of the AIDS Task Force, has claimed that the hidden agenda behind the safe-sex campaign is protection of the 'fast-lane' lifestyles of homosexuals. Pennington has argued that playing down the fact that homosexual sex is statistically *far* more likely to lead to Human Immunodeficiency Virus (HIV) infection than heterosexual sex, and arguing that everyone is at risk and should therefore adopt the safe-sex guidlines, simply deflects attention from the fact that homosexual men who are infected with the virus have an obligation to curtail their activities so as not to place others at risk.

This book seeks to provide a dispassionate analysis of some problems generated by AIDS. It covers the basic medical facts, some ethical and legal issues, and information on how to protect oneself from the risk of becoming HIV infected. It also sets out an argument which justifies the move from ethics to discriminatory public policies, and addresses the particular problems raised by AIDS in schools, prisons, the intravenous drug using community, and sexual relationships.

I will argue that while AIDS may appear to be unique, this appearance is deceptive. Infection with the AIDS virus is just one of many risks faced by individuals within our society. There are numerous other risks to health and life we all face every day — for example, one places both oneself and others at risk whenever one drives down a suburban street.

Society is prepared to countenance some risks, but not others. Individuals are permitted to drive motor vehicles but only if they are licensed, and provided they observe the road rules and speed limits. In the case of AIDS, the fundamental question requiring an answer is: where is the boundary which divides acceptable from unacceptable risk? In the following chapters I shall attempt to answer this important question.

1 THE MEDICAL FACTS

Acquired Immune Deficiency Syndrome (AIDS) is a very serious, indeed deadly disease. AIDS was 'discovered' in the wake of increasing reports from California and New York City of the unusual occurrence of life-threatening opportunistic infections and Kaposi's sarcoma in young, previously healthy, homosexual males. The former category — that of the opportunistic infection — is a category of illnesses which are not usually found or, if found, are found in relatively mild forms in people with normal immune systems.

An opportunistic infection is one where the infection occurs while the patient is undergoing some treatment and where that treatment predisposes the patient toward the acquiring of the infection. Prior to the AIDS epidemic Pneumocystis pneumonia and Kaposi's sarcoma were sometimes found in organ transplant patients whose immune defences had been suppressed by drugs used to prevent rejection of the newly grafted organ. But with AIDS, the infections in question do not arise as the result of drug treatments. These infections are classified as opportunistic only because they *resemble* the infections suffered by individuals whose immune systems have been suppressed by the administration of drugs.

OPPORTUNISTIC INFECTIONS ASSOCIATED WITH AIDS

Kaposi's sarcoma is a rare form of cancer. More specifically, it is a malignant tumour of the connective tissues that appears as ugly purplish-pink spots on the skin. In some cases this sarcoma assumes a virulent form which attacks other organs. It may infect the lungs, making breathing difficult, or cause heavy bleeding in the bowel. It may also attack the bones, causing them to crack, thus releasing calcium into the bloodstream — a condition which causes the patient severe pain.

Pneumosystis pneumonia is an inflammation of the lungs. The

patient experiences chest pain, coughing, high fever and breathing difficulties. All these become acute in the latter stages of the illness as the patient suffers rapid weight loss, and severe fatigue.

Toxoplasmosis gondii and Candida albicans also occur frequently in AIDS patients. The toxoplasmosis virus can attack all organs of the body. In the brain it causes encephalitis with concomitant headaches, dizziness and confusion. It may also attack the heart muscles and make the patient more vulnerable to heart attack. Candida albicans — otherwise known as thrush — may be so thick in the mouths and throats of AIDS patients that swallowing becomes very difficult and sometimes impossible.

Cryptococcus Neoformans lodges principally in the meninges, the membranes which enclose the brain and spinal cord. The patient suffers headaches and has difficulty focusing. He or she becomes confused and depressed and loses the ability to speak coherently.

Cytomegalovirus and Epstein-Barr virus are both members of the herpes virus family. In an immuno-supressed individual cytomegalovirus can be lethal, causing hepatitis and pneumonia. The Epstein-Barr virus is responsible for mononucleosis (glandular fever), again a condition that is not usually serious, but can become so in an immuno-suppressed individual.

Patients with AIDS typically fall victim to more than one of these serious illnesses. By the time they die they are both wasted and disfigured. For the doctors treating them there is the constant demoralisation of patients who on first presentation look relatively normal, but within a year are wizened and on the verge of death.

AIDS RELATED COMPLEX

AIDS Related Complex (or ARC) is another manifestation of HIV infection. Though it may be serious, ARC is not necessarily fatal. Those who have it do not suffer from the opportunistic infections and cancers associated with AIDS, but they are subject to fevers, night sweats, enlarged lymph nodes in neck, armpits and groin, unexplained weight loss, diarrhoea, persistent cough, oral thrush, shingles, fatigue and loss of appetite.

A significant proportion of those with ARC go on to develop AIDS.

ASYMPTOMATIC HIV INFECTION

Finally there are those who are infected with the HIV (or AIDS) virus but have no symptoms. These individuals comprise the largest group of those infected with HIV. We cannot be sure how many individuals are so infected but the National Health and Medical Research Council Special Unit in AIDS Epidemiology and Clinical Research estimates that between 12 000 and 13 000 Australians have had a positive result to the HIV antibody test, and that the total number of people infected with the HIV virus is of the order of 50 000. All of these 50 000 individuals are capable of transmitting the virus to others and a large number of them can be expected to go on to develop AIDS or ARC.

AIDS IN THE BRAIN

Although most attention to date has focused on HIV's effects on the immune system, the virus also has dramatic direct effects on the central nervous system. These effects are not opportunistic. They are quite distinct from the abscesses and tumours of the brain that occur as a result of damage to the immune system.

When the HIV virus attacks the brain directly it causes lesions within the white matter of that organ. The patient may in consequence suffer dementia, violent mood swings, speech and coordination difficulties or mimic any one of a number of other neurological syndromes from multiple sclerosis to schizophrenia. Some experts believe that, in time, these neurological consequences will overshadow the immunological ones. The fact that the HIV virus is able to cross the blood-brain barrier into the brain is particularly disturbing because most anti-viral agents are unable to do so.

CLASSIFICATION OF HIV INFECTIONS

How are we to classify the different manifestations of infection with the HIV virus? The most serious cases are those where individuals have full-blown AIDS. This is frequently referred to as AIDS category A, or just plain AIDS. AIDS category B includes individuals with Lymphadenopathy Syndrome (LAS), and those with other symptoms which constitute what is referred to as the AIDS Related Complex or ARC. AIDS category C includes individuals who have a confirmed antibody positive test result for the HIV virus, but have no symptoms (i.e. they are quite healthy). And then of course there are individuals who have been infected with the virus, but have not had an antibody test, or have had an antibody test that was negative because the antibodies had not had sufficient time to develop.

WHAT CAUSES AIDS?

AIDS is caused by a virus, or more specifically the Human Immunodeficiency Virus type I, (HIV). Credit for the discovery of this virus is shared by French and American scientists. At the Pasteur Institute in Paris in 1983 a group of French scientists headed by Luc Montagnier succeeded in isolating a strain of the virus which causes AIDS. An American group headed by Robert Gallo isolated another strain in 1984. The HIV virus is also sometimes referred to as HTLV III (Human T-cell Lymphatropic Virus type III), or LAV (Lymphadenopathy Associated Virus). A decision to refer to the AIDS virus as HIV came in the wake of considerable controversy over the question of who first discovered it, and was motivated by considerations of diplomacy. Prior to this whether one referred to it as HTLV III or LAV was determined primarily by one's nationality (HTLV III if you were American, LAV if you were French!).

WHERE DID AIDS COME FROM?

There were numerous early theories about the cause of AIDS. It was suggested that the disease was caused by 'poppers' — amyl nitrate — taken by homosexuals to enhance sexual pleasure. Others thought it was caused by an overload to the immune system — more specifically by repeated exposure to sperm, other foreign proteins or infectious agents. Some even suggested it was caused by organisms that had escaped from biological warfare laboratories, or, more insidiously, by organisms released in the United States by agents of the USSR.

Another (and more down to earth) theory claimed that the AIDS virus may have mutated from a similar virus found in the African Green Monkey. The latter virus — Simion T-Lymphotrophic Virus type III (STLV-III) — does not usually cause disease in the Green Monkey but, according to this theory, it may have undergone mutation in human beings to become the AIDS virus. The major objection raised against this proposal at the time when the theory was first advanced was that the HIV and STLV-III viruses were not sufficiently closely related.

More recently, however, the theory has gained support from the discovery of a group of intermediate viruses. One of these, the HTLV-IV virus, was isolated in West Africa in 1985. It is closely related to STLV-III and it infects human beings without usually causing disease. A plausible hypothesis is that STLV-III entered the human population (possibly from monkey bites), initiating a series of mutations which resulted in the HIV (or AIDS) virus.

TRANSMISSION

The AIDS virus has been found in all bodily fluids (precious and otherwise): blood, urine, semen, saliva, and even tear drops. This is at first sight alarming. And not surprisingly the discovery of the virus in saliva prompted a good deal of public alarm. The US Fire Brigades Union, for example, instructed its members not to offer mouth to mouth resuscitation to anyone they suspected of being homosexual.

But there is no evidence that the virus is transmitted via saliva in casual contacts. Nor is it spread via swimming pools or toilet seats or by handshakes or hugs. There is no evidence that it is spread through food, water or air. On the contrary, the transmission of the HIV virus requires close personal contact. It is transmitted through sexual contacts involving exchanges of body fluids, and through contaminated blood, blood products and hypodermics.

Because of this mode of transmission, the AIDS virus is importantly different from the various flu viruses which are frequently transmitted via aerosols of infected saliva. A virus (any virus) can infect a person only by first entering the cells of that person's body. This is because a virus is *entirely dependent* upon the enzymes in living cells for its own reproduction. A virus can enter the body by either infecting a cell on one of the surfaces, external or internal, or by infecting a non-surface cell after some trauma.

The surfaces of the respiratory and gastrointestinal tracts are particularly vulnerable to viruses because they are designed to absorb oxygen, food and water from the environment. Measles, influenza and the common cold are all caused by viruses which leave the body in invisible droplets when an infected person sneezes. Another individual in the vicinity breathes in some of the droplets, which attach to and multiply within the cells lining the respiratory tract. Hepatitis B virus (Serum Hepatitis), on the other hand, is unable to multiply within any epithelial cell. It requires a breach in the body surface to get it into the blood stream where it may then be carried to the liver.

In the West, AIDS was first diagnosed among members of the gay community. The other groups at particular risk were soon recognised as being intravenous drug-users and haemophiliacs. AIDS, it seemed, had a transmission pattern similar to that of Hepatitis B: it was not transmissible through epithelial cells but had to be introduced directly into the bloodstream. In the case of homosexuals the introduction of the virus into the bloodstream was achieved as a result of anal intercourse — a practice which frequently leads to tears in the rectal wall. Intravenous drug users and haemophiliacs became infected because the virus had been pumped directly into their veins.

The HIV virus is a retrovirus. What this means is that, unlike most other viruses, HIV changes the structure of the cells it attacks. When the HIV virus infects a cell, its genetic code becomes incorporated in the code of that cell. When the cell multiplies it then automatically produces more virus. One consequence of HIV being a retrovirus is that there is no way of getting rid of the virus without getting rid of its host cell. Put more bluntly this means that people infected with HIV will remain infected for life.

The HIV virus undermines the human immune system by killing a group of white blood cells known as the T-helper (or T4) cells. These T-helper cells usually play a vital role in preventing infection. When an infection occurs they do two things. First, they signal to other parts of the immune system that an infection has occurred, and the body responds by producing antibodies to fight the infectious agent. Second, the T-helper cells signal to another group of white blood cells — the T-suppressor (or T-8) cells — when it is time for the immune system to cease activities. In people with normal immune systems the ratio of T-helper to T-suppressor cells is 2:1. In people with AIDS that ratio is reversed. As a result of this a person with AIDS has fewer T-helper cells to fight infection, while the T-suppressor cells work to prevent what helper cells there are from doing their job. The person with AIDS is left defenceless against infection.

AIDS IN AFRICA

In Africa infection with HIV appears to be far more widespread than in the West. Some estimate that between five and ten million Africans living in the central tropical zone may already be infected with the virus. And the occurrence of AIDS in Africa displays a pattern quite unlike that in the United States. In Africa AIDS affects men and women in almost equal numbers (Hancock and Carim, 1986: 123). Various hypotheses have been advanced in explanation of this striking difference. Some have suggested that the African practice of reusing 'disposable' needles might provide an explanation. Others have suggested that heterosexual anal intercourse may be more prevalent in Africa than in the United States. As yet, however, no consensus has been reached with respect to the answer to this puzzle.

It now appears that a second type of AIDS virus is spreading from Africa into the West. In 1986 a new human retrovirus — HIV II — was isolated in persons from West Africa. As yet, little is known about HIV II, apart from the fact that like HIV it causes immunodeficiency and AIDS. But the discovery of HIV II must raise the question of the possibility of there being even more variants of the HIV virus. At a more prosaic level the existence of HIV II raises problems with respect to ensuring the purity of the blood supply, since ten per cent of cases of HIV II infection are undetectable by the currently available antibody screening kits. Scientists are presently working on developing a second antibody test kit that will pick up this ten per cent.

THE PROGNOSIS

The prognosis for individuals infected with the HIV virus is far from rosy. As the disease has been monitored only since 1981 definitive pronouncements are still not possible. Using the data acquired during the first three years of monitoring it was estimated that within three years of infection five to fifteen per cent of people would develop AIDS, and another 25 to 35 per cent ARC (Gust, 1985: 10). But it was pointed out, even at that time, that it would be unrealistic to expect these figures to go down as time went by and more data was acquired.

More recent estimates made by the World Health Organization put the probability of developing AIDS within five years of infection at between ten and 30 per cent, and the probability of developing ARC at between 20 and 50 per cent. A new six stage classification of HIV infection has been developed by Robert R. Redfield of the Walter Reid Army Institute of Research. Redfield has used this classification to follow a group of patients for 36 months. He found that about 90 per cent of them progressed to a more serious stage (Gallo, 1987: 47-8). These results suggest that there may be very few individuals who remain permanently without symptoms. Maybe everyone infected with the virus will eventually succumb to the disease.

One of the enigmas presented by AIDS (and infectious diseases generally) is the fact that some individuals are more susceptible to infection than others. A recent British study has identified genetic combinations which appear to bestow greater and lesser susceptibility to infection by the HIV virus (*The Economist* 23 May, 1987: 89-90). This would explain why some individuals have not contracted the virus even though participating in regular unprotected anal sex with infected partners. It would also explain why some infected individuals develop symptoms more quickly than others. But while there may be a large degree of variation among individuals between the time of infection and the development of symptoms, recent results suggest that very few (if any) infected individuals can expect to remain well. It is simply of matter of time.

DETECTION OF THE PRESENCE OF HIV

Once it was known that HIV virus could be passed on via blood and blood products, a high priority was to find a means for ensuring the purity of the blood supply. The first and obvious way to promote this end was to discourage individuals at risk from donating (or in the USA, selling) their blood.

Australia now requires all blood donors to both sign a declaration to the effect that they do not belong to any group which is at high risk for infection with the HIV virus, and to have an HIV antibody test. Individuals who make misleading declarations are liable to legal penalties which may involve both fines and imprisonment.

The probability of being infected with HIV as the result of a blood transfusion is now believed to be very low. Problems, however, remain. In the first place, there are individuals who do not believe they belong to a risk category, but nevertheless do. The wives of bisexual men and the spouses of intravenous drug-users are obvious examples. There may also be a few individuals who recklessly or maliciously continue to donate blood while knowing that they belong to a risk category.

The USA experiences these problems plus an additional one. Since one may sell one's blood in the US, there is a monetary incentive for individuals at risk to go ahead, regardless of the harm they may cause to others. Intravenous drug users clearly fall within this category. There already is a very high risk that one will contract Hepatitis B if transfused with commercially procured blood. This is because many intravenous drug users will sell their blood as a means of raising cash.

The antibody screening tests currently used within Australia are the ELISA (Enzyme-Linked Immunosorbent Assays) and the Western Blot. The procedure employed is to first use an ELISA. If the result is positive, a second ELISA is used. If the result is still positive the blood is then subjected to the Western Blot, which is both a more complex and more expensive procedure for looking at the same reaction.

Since no antibody test is perfect there will be some individuals whose results are positive, while they do not actually have any HIV virus within their blood. Such results are referred to as false positives. A false positive is not much fun for the individual who has tested positive. However with respect to securing the purity of the blood supply these false positives are unproblematic. It is rather the false negatives — individuals who test antibody negative but who have been infected with the HIV virus — that are the problem.

The incidence of false negatives using the ELISA is believed to be low. But there are some false negatives, and these occur, for the most part, because the individual has his or her antibody test before sufficient time has elapsed for antibodies to the HIV virus to develop. The development of antibodies may take up to nine weeks. So if individuals donate blood between the time of infection with the HIV virus and the development of antibodies they will test negative even though they are infected with the virus.

An obvious suggestion at this point is that the blood be kept for nine weeks and then tested. But while this is feasible in the case of some blood products, it is not possible in the case of red blood cells. It is these red blood cells that most transfused individuals need but, unfortunately, unless blood is used within three weeks all the red blood cells are dead. Interestingly, the HIV virus does not infect the red blood cells. However it is not possible to 'wash' them completely free of virus.

A good antibody test has both high specificity and high sensitivity. Its sensitivity is good to the extent that it picks up *all* cases where the relevant antibody is present. Its specificity is good to the extent that it *only* picks up cases where the relevant antibody is present. Unfortunately no real antibody tests are perfect. The ELISA is good as these things go. The Western Blot is even better. But they are not perfect.

As things stand at present there are two threats to the purity of the blood supply. The first is posed by those individuals who believe they do not belong to any high risk group but in fact do. The second is posed by the HIV II virus. As yet we do not know the extent of the spread of this virus beyond Africa. But we do know that our present screening tests, developed to detect antibodies to the HIV virus, fail to pick up antibodies to HIV II in about ten per cent of the tested cases.

ADDITIONAL READING

Black, D. *The Plague Years* London: Picador, 1986

Brass, A. and Gold, J. *AIDS and Australia* Sydney: Bay Books, 1985

The Economist, 'Why some people get AIDS and others don't' 23 May, 1987

Gallo, R. C. 'The First Human Retrovirus' *Scientific American* December, 1986

Gallo, R. C. 'The AIDS Virus' *Scientific American* January, 1987

Gust, I.D., 'AIDS' *Bioethics News* Vol. 5, No. 1, 1985

Hancock, G. and Carim, E. *AIDS: The Deadly Epidemic* London: Gollancz, 1986

Mann, J. 'The Global Strategy for AIDS Prevention and Control' Geneva: The World Health Organisation, 5 May, 1987

QUESTIONS

1 What is AIDS?
2 What are the symptoms of AIDS category A?
3 What are the symptoms of AIDS category B?
4 What are the symptoms of AIDS category C?
5 Why is it a problem to have AIDS category C?
6 If Fred has an AIDS antibody test and the result is negative what does this show?
7 If Mary has an AIDS antibody test and the result is positive what does this show?
8 How is the AIDS virus passed from one person to another?
9 List some activities that would put a person at high risk of contracting AIDS.
10 List some of the myths about contracting AIDS — ways you will not catch AIDS.

2   Ethics

MARY: I've had enough! Jim's top of the class again for that history assignment. And he sat there looking so smug!

JILL: What makes it worse is that he thinks he's putting it over us. I've a mind to let him know otherwise. He's not the only one with an older brother doing history at the uni.

JANE: Yes, but your brother isn't prepared to give you essays to copy. And if he did, can you really say you wouldn't copy?

JILL: I certainly hope I wouldn't. But suppose I did — that wouldn't make it right. It would just mean I'd sunk as low as Jim.

MARY: Well, I know I wouldn't. I couldn't. It's wrong to steal someone else's work and then pass it off as your own.

JANE: I suppose it is. But, you know, sometimes I have my doubts. After all, maybe it's just showing a bit of initiative. I don't believe all these history assignments are really good for us. And I bet lots of kids in this school cheat. You'd be a fool not to, when so much of our HSC mark is made up by internal assessment. Why shouldn't we all use any tactic we can to get the best mark possible?

JILL: But imagine if that is how everyone behaved, Jane. Suppose everyone did whatever he or she could get away with in any kind of situation — and with respect to things far more serious than history exams. Society would fall apart. The only reason it holds together is because most people are prepared to do the right thing most of the time.

MARY: That's beside the point. Cheating on an assignment is wrong because it's stealing someone else's work. Period.

ETHICS 13

JILL: But there's more to it than that, Mary. Stealing may mostly be wrong. But was it wrong for prisoners of war to steal from their guards when they were starving? Lying may mostly be wrong but is it wrong to lie to protect someone or tell a white lie to make your grandmother happy? I think it's much more complicated.

DEBBIE: I think all morality is relative. After all, the Iranians think it's okay to stone a woman if she commits adultery, and we think that's wrong. You can't prove it one way or the other.

MARY: Well, I for one sure don't agree with that, Debbie. And neither does Jill or Jane, judging by the looks on their faces. The case of the Iranians just shows that it's possible for a whole society to be wrong about something.

DEBBIE: But you can't prove it.

JILL: I can, because once you accept that the morally right action is the one that produces more happiness, it's clear that they are wrong, whatever they think.

DEBBIE: But suppose those doing the stoning get more happiness out of it than the woman would if she were let off. Would that change your position, Jill?

JILL: Well, I have to admit that is a bit of a problem for me.

MARY: And Jill, you'd also have to say that slavery was okay, so long as there was more happiness overall with slavery than without it.

JILL: That seems a bit improbable given how many slaves there were and how they were treated. But I take your point.

JANE: But Mary, I can't see how your view is any better. You say it's wrong to steal someone else's ideas and I supose you'd say it was wrong to make someone a slave because...

MARY: Because people have rights. They have rights to liberty and to their ideas and to all sorts of things. Slavery and stealing are wrong because they interfere with those rights.

JANE: But how can you show what rights there are? And more importantly, how can you solve difficulties which arise when rights come into collision? If morality is the way you describe it then there is no experiment we can perform to discover what is really right and wrong.

DEBBIE: So it's just relative!

JANE: No, I don't think that follows.

MARY: What do you think, Jane?

JANE: I suppose I think that we all have an instinct to survive as best we can. Therefore it's right to do whatever one needs to survive and get on in the world.

MARY: Even if you can only get on by killing your boss?

JANE: Well, no, because you'd be likely to be caught and sent to prison. That wouldn't be in your best interest.

MARY: But if there were no chance of being caught?

JANE: I suppose I have to say it's okay.

JILL: But Jane, that's not morality, that's just self-interest!

Ethics is about right and wrong. But then, what *makes* some actions right and others wrong? Is an action right because it accords with a rule of conduct, or is it right because it gives rise to better consequences than its alternative? Or is it right for some other reason? In this chapter we will look at some of the ways that philosophers — both living and dead — have attemped to answer this question. But first let's clarify one or two points. In ordinary conversation the terms 'moral' and 'ethical' are frequently used as synonyms for 'morally good' or 'morally right'. Philosophers do not use them in such a way. For philosophers, an individual is behaving morally if he or she is behaving in accordance with some set of ethical (moral) standards. It is not required that the standards be the correct ones, or even the ones commonly accepted within the individual's community.

So there are really two interesting questions. First there is the general question of what criteria a set of standards must satisfy before they may be seen as constitutive of a morality. The second question is the question of which morality (if any) is *the* correct one.

Looking at something as abstract as the nature of morality in this way allows us to make some important distinctions. First there is the distinction between moral and amoral behaviour — that is, behaviour governed by some set of moral standards and behaviour governed by no such standards. And, given the assumption that there is some correct ethical view, it also allows us to classify some actions as well-intentioned but wrong. Suppose, for the sake of argument, that abortion is wrong according to *the* correct ethical theory. Wendy Louise, who subscribes to another system of ethics, believes it is right for her, given her circumstances, to have an abortion. She has one. We may now say that what she did is objectively wrong, but still allow that she is a good person because she did what she believed to be right (that is, she behaved in accordance with the principles of *her* ethical system).

ARE THERE ANY FEATURES THAT AN ETHICAL THEORY *MUST* HAVE?

Philosophers agree that a person who acts according to some set of ethical standards will be able to offer some justification for his or her actions. However, a justification in terms of self-interest alone will not do. It cannot be right for me to do something, and wrong for you to do that very same thing. Moral principles must be formulable in a way that prescribes that *any* individual who satisfies certain general criteria should behave in a given way. For example, I cannot argue that it is wrong for you to steal a car, but not wrong for me to steal a car simply because it suits me to have a car I did not have to pay for.

Of course there may be circumstances in which it may be right for an individual to 'steal' a car. Imagine that Fred and Joe are driving down a deserted highway when they collide with another vehicle. The driver of the second vehicle is thrown from the wreck and killed. Joe is seriously injured and bleeding heavily. Fred and Joe's car is destroyed and will not start. So Fred 'steals' the other vehicle to drive the bleeding Joe to the nearest town and medical assistance. Here it is right for Fred to 'steal' the car. But it would also be right for anyone else faced with the same situation to do the same thing.

ETHICAL EGOISM

According to ethical egoism each individual has one, and only one, basic obligation, which is to bring about for himself or herself the greatest possible balance of good consequences over bad, or utility over disutility. Utility is a general term frequently used in economic literature to refer to good or pleasant consequences. Gains in income, job promotions, happy love affairs are the kinds of things that typically increase utility. Disutility, on the other hand, is a general term for referring to bad or unpleasant consequences. Sickness, the death of a friend, and loss of one's job all typically serve to increase disutility.

The ethical egoist allows that each of us is entitled to act in a way that promotes his or her own best interests. But an individual is not required to make the same moral assessment of an action regardless of whether or not he himself benefits or suffers as a result of that action. For example, the ethical egoist can claim it is (morally) right for he himself to defraud his company when there is little chance that he will be caught. At the same time that person can claim it is (morally) wrong for another director to do the same thing.

It is this feature which disqualifies ethical egoism from being a true moral theory. Ethical egoism is just self-interest disguised as morality.

RELATIVISM IN ETHICS

Many modern individuals argue that what is right or wrong is only right or wrong relative to the society in which one lives. According to such a view it is wrong for an Australian to stone a woman because she has commited adultery, but it is not wrong for an Iranian to do so. The cultures are different, the moralities are different, and so an action that is morally wrong in one culture may be morally right in another. For the relativist, differing moral evaluations of a particular action are justified in terms of the action taking place in different societies with different conventions.

It is not necessary to look far to see a crushing objection to relativism. Take, for example, the institution of slavery. According to the relativist, a non-conformist who lives in a society where slavery is an acceptable institution is simply wrong when he or she argues that slavery is morally wrong. However, if the non-conformist can convert a sufficient number of others to his or her view, then slavery will become morally wrong. Similarly, if it had been the case that more than 50 per cent of the population in Nazi Germany considered it morally correct to exterminate the Jews, then indeed, according to the relativist, it would have been morally right at that time in that society to exterminate the Jews.

Any moral theory committed to results like these lacks plausibility.

SUBJECTIVISM

Another approach frequently taken to ethical questions is to claim that ethical judgements are merely subjective. According to this view there need be no fact of the matter as to whether rape is right or wrong. In claiming that it is wrong an individual is merely voicing his or her negative attitude toward it. But another individual may have a positive attitude toward it and for that individual it need not be wrong. Take Bill. He is a viscious thug and considers it his right to have sex with any woman he desires, whether or not she agrees to be a party to it. Mary Lou refuses to have sex with Bill and so Bill rapes her. Later he claims that he has done nothing morally wrong. Indeed he argues that since Mary Lou refused him and he felt entitled to have sex with her, there was nothing he could do but force her to submit. And, according to the subjectivist, if Bill is speaking the truth then he has indeed done what is morally right for him.

If one accepts the subjectivist's view one must accept that any ethical judgement is as good as any other so long as it expresses the genuine attitude of the agent. What is more, all arguments then become irrelevant. Why argue about ethical judgements when the one is already as good as the other?

RULES AND RIGHTS

A moral system with which most of us are familiar and one which provides us with a set of rules to follow is that contained in Christianity. These rules are the Ten Commandments, which most Christians (and Jews) believe should be followed because they are the commands of God.

Those who, upon consideration of the evidence, do not believe that God exists must obviously be sceptical of an ethical theory grounded on what are purported to be commands of God. But even if one does accept that God exists, it may still be argued, as it was by Plato two thousand years ago, that what makes the commands of God correct moral principles is not simply the fact that they are God's commands. Suppose God were to command us to torture some five-year-old child. That God has made this command would not make what we did morally correct.

Plato suggests that God has given us certain commands because what the commands urge us to do is independently morally correct. But then we are left with our original problem: what is it that make some actions morally good and others morally bad?

The seventeenth century English philosopher John Locke was one who attempted to answer this question. Locke argued that men possess certain natural rights — the rights to life, health, liberty and property. In Locke's view an individual does something morally wrong when he or she interferes with that to which another has a right. If I murder a man or steal his car I do something morally wrong.

But was Locke correct when he argued that all men possess the rights to life, health, liberty and property? At first glance most of us would want to agree that each of us has these rights. But even rights so seemingly basic as these become problematic upon closer inspection. Sure, I have a right to life. But suppose I have no money and no food. Does this mean that the state has a duty to supply me with these things? Some believe this to be so, others do not. The Libertarian, for example, believes that it is wrong to take money, by taxation, from some individuals to provide for the needs of others. He argues that this constitutes an unjustifiable interference with the liberty of the taxed individuals.

And does the foetus have a right to life? The Right To Life group claim that it does. But there are also those who disagree. Some argue that forcing a woman to bear a child she does not want is an unjustifiable interference with her liberty. Others argue that the foetus is not a person and so has no right to life.

Whatever else it may be, the foetus is certainly a member of the species *Homo sapiens*, albeit a very young one. Those who claim it is not a person make a distinction between being a person and being a member of the species *Homo sapiens* — that is, being a human being. They argue that an individual is only a person if it has fairly sophisticated beliefs and desires and is conscious of itself as having a future. The foetus is not such an individual. Therefore it is not a person, and therefore it has no right to life.

But another consequence of arguing that only persons have a right to life is that it now seems that the severely demented, the severely retarded and those in comas do not have a right to life. And while many are prepared to accept abortion, far fewer are prepared to accept that killing the severely retarded or demented is morally justified.

Now the right to property. Again there has been much debate throughout history as to whether individuals have any such right. Capitalism is predicated upon the assumption that individuals have this right, and socialism upon the assumption that there is no such right.

Some philosophers talk about duties rather than rights, but this amounts to much the same thing. In general it is true that my having a right to something means that you have a corresponding duty not to interfere with my right. If I own a car I have a right to it, and you have a corresponding duty not to steal it.

A general problem with rules, rights and duties is that it is impossible to formulate a rule which admits of no exceptions. Take, for example, the rule: Be truthful. What is one to do if asked by a violent husband, 'Where is my wife hiding?' In reply to this kind of objection some philosophers distinguish *prima facie* duties from actual ones. One always has a *prima facie* duty to be truthful, but when faced with a conflict of duties of the kind just outlined one's *actual* duty may involve telling a lie.

But how can one tell when one should tell a lie? More generally, how can one tell what is one's actual duty when one is faced with a conflict of duties? I promise to visit my sick friend in hospital but then I realise I have also promised to mow the lawn of the old lady next door. What should I do? Which is my actual or *real* duty?

The problem of producing a hierarchical ordering of duties or rights is avoidable if one has only one duty or right. Take the Golden Rule of the Bible, 'Do unto others as you would have them do unto you'. What is wrong with the Golden Rule is that it leaves the individual as the arbiter of right and wrong. What one individual would do in some situation of moral decision may be quite different from what another individual would do. A man coming from a wealthy background who has not been successful may sincerely believe that his lack of success is due to the fact that he was never forced to be self-reliant. His son, down on his luck, asks for help. The father refuses to help him, genuinely believing that this is the right thing to do. He has applied the Golden Rule, and this is what he wishes his father had done for him when he was in the same position. A second man believes his unsuccessful life is due to the fact that his father did not lend him financial assistance when he was young and in need. His son comes to him for help and he willingly gives it. He has applied the Golden Rule and this is what he wishes his father had done.

Each of these two men has applied the Golden Rule to the same problem but come up with a different answer, which shows that the Golden Rule cannot provide us with an objective standard of morality.

IMMANUEL KANT

The eighteenth century German philosopher Immanuel Kant propounded a view which is able to avoid this problem of non-objectivity. Kant argued that each individual should act in that way which he or she could will all other individuals faced with the same decision to act. Kant's famous categorical imperative states that an individual should, 'Act only on that maxim through which you can at the same time will that it become a universal law.'

On first inspection Kant's position sounds rather similar to the Golden Rule we have just discussed. But there is one important difference. According to Kant's view, the way an individual should act is not how any actual flesh and blood individual would choose to act but rather how a perfectly rational individual would act. And how would such a perfectly rational individual act? Let's look at an example discussed by Kant, that of making deceitful promises. Suppose I promise my friend that I will meet her at a restaurant at a given time, fully intending that if I get a better offer in the meantime I will not show up. Kant argues that to make this promise, while at the same time intending to break the promise if certain contingencies eventuate, is not something that the perfectly rational individual could will to become a universal law — that is, it is not something which can satisify his categorical imperative.

Kant's reason for saying this is not, as one might expect, that the consequences of everyone breaking their promises when it suited them would be very bad. Rather it is that one would be involved in a contradiction if one were to will as a universal law that individuals be able both to make a promise and have that promise believed, and at the same time everyone be free to break promises whenever it suited their purposes. Put less formally, what Kant is saying is that promising is only possible because an expectation exists that individuals will honour their promises, even though honouring a promise may not be the most convenient thing to do. For similar reasons Kant holds that it is always wrong to lie. For how can one expect to be believed when one makes a statement if everyone also accepts that whenever it is to an individual's advantage to lie he or she will do so?

What about those occasions when lying would produce far better results than telling the truth? What should one do when asked by a violent husband, 'Where is my wife hiding?' According to Kant one is still obligated to tell the truth. The fact that telling the truth in this case will result in far worse consequences than telling a lie is irrelevant to Kant. Kant is self-avowedly not interested in consequences. Indeed he believes that worrying about consequences will often have pernicious results.

But how could I *ever* be in a position to will that my action become a universal law if I do not take serious stock of the consequences of that action and its alternatives? It seems that one *has* to look at consequences in order to be able to make a decision that one would have adequate grounds for being able to will as a universal law.

JOHN RAWLS

The contemporary American philosopher John Rawls offers an account of morality which is, according to his own estimation, fundamentally Kantian. Kant argues that the morally right action is the action that a perfectly rational individual would choose. But, as we have seen, it seems impossible for such a perfectly rational agent to have adequate grounds for willing his action to become a universal law if he does not examine the consequences of the alternative actions open to him.

Rawls' solution to the problem of deciding what is right and what is wrong is to argue that our fundamental ethical principles are those we would select to maximise our long-run utility if we were to make the selection from behind a 'veil of ignorance'. This veil obscures from the individual the actual abilities and material benefits he or she is to have. The individual does not know whether he will be born poor or rich, male or female, intelligent or stupid.

> The idea of the original position is to set up a fair procedure so that any principles agreed to will be just. ... Somehow we must nullify the effects of specific contingencies which put men at odds and tempt them to exploit social and natural circumstances to their own advantage. Now in order to do this I assume that the parties are situated behind a veil of ignorance. They do not know how the various alternatives will effect their own particular case and they are obliged to evaluate principles solely on the basis of general considerations. ... It is assumed, then, that the parties do not know various kinds of particular facts. First of all no one knows his place in society, his class position or social status; nor does he know his conception of the good, the particulars of his rational plan of life, or even the special features of his psychology such as his aversion to risk or liability to optimism or pessimism. ... The persons in the original position have no information as to which generation they belong. ... As far as possible then the

only particular facts which the parties know is that their society is subject to the circumstances of justice and whatever that implies. It is taken for granted, however, that they know the general facts about human society. They understand political affairs and the principles of economic theory; they know the basis of social organization and the laws of human psychology. (Rawls, 1972: 136-7)

By using the 'veil of ignorance' device individuals are prevented from choosing their fundamental ethical principles on the basis of sectional interests, for the veil obscures whether they will be the ones to gain or lose by the principles they select. Like the ethical egoist, Rawls selects his principles on the basis of the ability of those principles to contribute to furthering the interests of the individual. But Rawls' theory is different from ethical egoism because Rawls' individuals have been stripped of all information about themselves. Unlike ethical egoism Rawls' theory cannot be accused of being self-interest disguised as ethics.

If we adopt the Rawlsian strategy for selecting ethical principles then our choice of principles will be determined by the expected consequences of those principles. Individuals behind the veil of ignorance will vote for those principles which can be expected to maximise their long-term interests. For example, they will vote for a rule which penalises individuals who steal because this rule can be expected to maximise the long-term interests of most members of the community — indeed, all of those who are not thieves. Each individual behind the veil of ignorance does not know whether or not he will be a thief. But given his knowledge of psychology and economics, he can assume that if there are sanctions against thieves the probability that he will not be a thief is far greater than the probability that he will be one. The absence of a rule penalising individuals who steal, on the other hand, could be expected to have very bad consequences for a community. If thieves are not penalised by the community then there will be no advantage to acquiring goods by honest toil, and so one would expect that in the long run more and more members of this community would abandon honest toil, which could be expected to lead to very serious consequences.

Rawls' strategy appears to be a good one for making decisions about the fundamental rules which should govern our societies.

But what of the more minor moral decisions all of us face in our everyday lives? Is the device of the veil of ignorance any real help in such situations? Maybe a simpler strategy would be adequate for such everyday purposes.

UTILITARIANISM

Like Rawls' theory, utilitarianism is concerned with consequences. For the utilitarian an action is right or wrong according to the consequences it generates. Jeremy Bentham, a classical utilitarian, argues that actions are right or wrong according to the pleasure or pain they give rise to. Peter Singer, a contemporary utilitarian, argues that furthering the interests of the individuals involved (and not simply increasing pleasure) is what a utilitarian should seek to do. John Stuart Mill, the best known utilitarian of all, has been interpreted in both of these ways.

Should I buy my sister a birthday present or give the money to the Salvation Army? According to the utilitarian, my decision should be determined by the consequences of these two possible actions. If I use the money to buy my sister a present she will feel happy because I have remembered her birthday and gone to the trouble of buying her a gift. But then some needy person in the care of the Salvation Army may have slightly less for lunch because of my decision. If I give the money to the Salvation Army there will be marginally more for lunch, but my sister will be hurt because she will feel unloved. So what should I do? According to the utilitarian, I should look at the consequences of each of these possible actions and then choose that action which has the better consequences.

Let's look at another, more serious, example. Fred is married to Jane and has two children, Bill and Sara. Fred also has a mistress Joan with whom he has been involved for some time. Fred is in love with Joan. Joan is in love with Fred. Should Fred leave Jane and move in with Joan? According to the utilitarian, the morally right decision is the one with the better consequences. If one is a Benthamite then one will be interested in the pleasure and pain generated by each of the two possible decisions. If one is an interest utilitarian rather than a Benthamite then what must be compared is how the interests of all those involved are effected by the two possible decisions. But in either case we must take into account the pleasures and pains, or interests, of *all* the individuals involved. Bill and Sara count just as much as Jane, Joan and Fred.

One objection often made against utilitarianism is that we cannot know for sure — that is, be 100 per cent certain — what the consequences of an action will be. Suppose Bob decides to lie to his mother about his whereabouts on Saturday afternoons. He tells her he is going roller skating but in fact he is having boxing lessons. He tells her this because she would worry if she knew the truth and he reasons that telling a lie will produce a better outcome. But one Saturday afternoon the skating rink catches fire. Bob's mother hears the news on the radio. Motoring toward the rink she fails to see a red light and is killed in a collision with a semi-trailer.

Bob did what he believed would produce the best consequences, but unfortunately a horrifying accident resulted from his lying. Opponents of utilitarianism may at this point argue that if Bob had done what, in their view, was the right thing — that is, told the truth — his mother would still be alive. In this case they would be correct.

Unfortunately, however, doing what is generally held to be the correct thing, or even behaving in a way that one might reasonably expect to produce the best results, does not always bring about those best results. Take Joe. Joe is also taking boxing lessons on Saturday afternoons. But unlike Bob he tells his mother the truth, though he knows this will cause her a lot of worry. Joe tells his mother he is having boxing lessons because he believes that the long run consequences of lying, and his mother discovering that he has lied, are so bad that it is better that she spend her Saturdays worrying.

Joe's mother spends Saturday afternoons in a state of agitation and distraction. One Saturday she is so preoccupied that she does not look before crossing the street and is knocked down and killed by a car.

Let us assume that both Bob and Joe are utilitarians and that each did what he believed would produce the best consequences. Unfortunately they were both wrong. With hindsight we can say that it would have been better if Joe had lied and Bob had told the truth. But the fact that it is possible to be wrong about the consequences of an action cannot absolve us from the responsibility of making the best estimate we can of the likely consequences of a particular action before we act. Maybe I'll be lucky and no one will be killed when I drive through my surburban shopping centre at 140 kph on a Saturday morning. But it is far more likely that someone will be injured. Like anyone else, the utilitarian cannot tell for certain what the future holds. The best he can do is work out what is most likely to happen and act accordingly.

Utilitarians divide into *act* and *rule* utilitarians. The act utilitarian is concerned with the consequences of each particular act. If it is the case that killing this innocent individual will result in the generation of more utility than letting him or her live, then according to act utilitarianism it is morally right to kill him or her.

But would it ever be reasonable to suppose that killing an innocent individual would result in better consequences than letting him or her live? Let's look at a hypothetical example. Suppose we have a community of blacks and whites where race relations are very bad. A white is killed and the white community believes that a black did it. But the person who did it cannot be found, and there is good reason to expect that if no one is arrested and executed for this crime many innocent blacks will be killed by the whites in retaliation. For the act utilitarian, detaining and killing an innocent black individual may be justified in these circumstances on the ground that it is preferable for one innocent individual to die rather than many.

Not surprisingly many find this consequence of act utilitarianism quite unacceptable, and therefore reject act utilitarianism. A fallback position is rule utilitarianism. According to this view one decides upon a set of moral rules according to their ability to increase utility. Then when one is faced with a particular decision, one simply applies the relevant rule. Killing the innocent can be excluded even for a rare exception like the hypothetical case described above, when such a killing would lead to the maximisation of utility. The rule utilitarian can argue that there should be a rule which prohibits killing the innocent, because to allow otherwise will produce greater disutility. If innocent individuals know that they may be killed merely to facilitate the general good they will live miserable, fearful lives. Overall, and in the long run, better consequences will be produced if there is a rule that the state does not allow the execution of innocent individuals. The rule utilitarian is a utilitarian only with respect to choosing his or her rules. In any particular situation of moral choice he or she makes no assessment of the consequences in that particular situation, he or she simply applies the relevant rule.

But is rule utilitarianism really any better than act utilitarianism? Suppose whites wish to live in white-only areas and there are very few blacks. In such a case it is arguable that the increased utility for the whites of being able to live in a white-only area may more than outweigh the disutility for the blacks when they are excluded from that area. And according to rule utilitarianism, segregation in such circumstances would be morally justified. But such a rule is deeply unjust, and so rule utilitarianism seems to be as unacceptable as act utilitarianism.

IN SUMMARY

I have traced a number of approaches to the solution of ethical problems and objections that may be made to them. Some are certainly more appealing than others. Subjectivism, Relativism and Ethical Egoism are all open to crushing objections. Although Utilitarianism, theories of rights and duties, the Golden Rule and the view of John Rawls have their problems too, all offer useful insights into the ethical questions we shall be discussing.

In the chapters which follow we shall be looking at some ethical issues thrown up by the phenomenon of AIDS. Questions like:

1 How should those who do not have AIDS or ARC, and who are not antibody positive, behave towards those who have AIDS, or ARC, or are antibody positive?
2 How should those who are antibody positive behave towards those who are not?
3 Should children who are antibody positive be able to attend schools?
4 To what extent should the resources of the community at large

be used to fund medical treatments for those suffering from AIDS or ARC?

What emerges is that the resolution of many of these issues will be the same whether one is a utilitarian, a rights theorist, a Kantian or an adherent to the Rawlsian view. This at first may seem surprising. But remember that the ethical philosopher is concerned primarily with giving an account of the nature of good and evil, so we might expect that alternative moral theories would agree about almost everything except the justifications they offer for their conclusions.

ADDITIONAL READING

Frankena, W. *Ethics* Englewood Cliffs, New Jersey: Prentice-Hall, 1963
Mill, J.S. 'Utilitarianism', in *Utilitarianism, Liberty, Representative Government* New York: Everyman, 1968
Plato, 'Euthyphro', *The Last Day of Socrates* London: Penguin,1969
Rachels, J. (ed.) *Moral Problems* New York: Harper and Row, 1975
Rawls, J. *A Theory of Justice* Oxford: Oxford University Press, 1972
Regan, T. (ed.) *Matters of Life and Death* New York: Random House, 1980
Singer, P. *Practical Ethics* Cambridge: Cambridge University Press, 1978
Singer, P. (ed.) *Applied Ethics* Oxford: Oxford University Press, 1986

QUESTIONS

1 'It is wrong to shoplift.'
   What would a utilitarian say about this?
   What would a rights theorist say?
   How about a subjectivist?
   How about a relativist?
   How about someone who was guided by the Golden Rule?
2 What are the dangers of accepting a moral theory which evaluates actions according to their consequences? What are the benefits?
3 Do you think people have any rights? What are they? What is the basis for claiming people have them?
4 Do you think animals have any rights? If your answer is yes, then what are they, and what is their basis? If your answer is no, explain why. If you answered yes to question (3) but no to this question explain why.

5 If there turned out to be intelligent beings on another planet would it be morally wrong to murder them or use them as slaves? Explain why, or why not. (Would how they looked be relevant? Would the kinds of minds they had be relevant?)
6 Imagine you are in Rawls' original position behind the veil of ignorance. From that position what would you have to say about:
   (a) regulating the use of alcohol, marijuana, heroin;
   (b) bigamous relationships (where a man has more than one wife or a woman more than one husband);
   (c) surrogate motherhood (where one woman pays another to have a child for her);
   (d) requiring people to have a licence to have children.

3 AIDS, Ethics and Sex

LONG-TERM SEXUAL RELATIONSHIPS

Case 1

Sue and David have been married for many years. Sue is a traditional housewife with conservative values. She believes that she is living within a monogamous relationship and her husband has encouraged this belief. But David, who is bisexual, also has casual homosexual relationships.

David, who like most of the rest of the community reads the paper and watches television, becomes aware of the fact that he may have been infected with the HIV virus. What is he to do? Confession to his wife could result in the collapse of their relationship. But if he says nothing and continues to have sexual relations with her she may be further exposed to the risk of infection.

Unfortunately for Sue, David is not a responsible person. He does nothing. He neither has an antibody test to find out whether he is infected with the HIV virus, nor does he tell her that he may possibly be infected and that she too therefore is at risk. But David is infected with the HIV virus. In time Sue too becomes infected.

One afternoon while shopping at the local mall Sue notices that the Red Cross Van is parked outside. She decides to make a blood donation. Sue knows that the government has asked all members of high risk groups to refrain from donating blood, and this has produced a situation where blood is in short supply. Sue signs the declaration that she does not belong to any risk group and makes her donation.

As regularly happens, the blood bank tests Sue's donation for HIV antibodies. The test is negative and so the blood goes off to a hospital where it is transfused into an accident victim, Bob, who has suffered severe blood loss. But unfortunately for Bob, Sue

AIDS, ETHICS AND SEX 31

is infected. She has not shown up as antibody positive because her infection has been very recent and so antibodies have not had time to develop. Her infected blood tranfused into Bob infects him too.

Sue is keen to have a baby. David is less enthusiastic but he has never been too careful about contraception. Sue always took responsibility for that. But now she wishes to be pregnant and so very soon she is. Pregnancy can accelerate the collapse of the immune system. And according to the World Health Organisation, a child born to an HIV infected mother has a 50 per cent chance of also being HIV infected. Of the babies so infected, more than half are dead within two years. Sue is unlucky, and both she and the baby she bears go on to develop AIDS. So too the unfortunate Bob.

Within five years, David, Sue, Bob and the baby are in the terminal stages of the disease. At least two and maybe three of these tragedies could have been avoided if David had behaved in a morally responsible manner and informed Sue that she was at risk when he realised that he himself might have been infected.

Case 2

Neil believes that he and Owen have had a monogamous relationship in the eight years they have lived together. Since Neil has never used intravenous drugs and is sure that Owen has not either he feels confident that he is not at risk of contracting AIDS.

But Owen, who regularly goes out of town on business, has used these occasions to shoot up with friends. Moreover, Owen has shared needles with these other friends. Since Neil strongly disapproves of drug use Owen has never told him that he is a user.

Owen knows about AIDS and that there is a high risk of becoming infected with HIV through sharing infected needles and unprotected anal intercourse. But he cannot face telling Neil that he has been an intravenous drug user and may be infected with the virus. So he just hopes that he has not been infected and goes on as usual.

Neil has a friend Sally who is 39 and has recently been divorced. Sally has decided that if she does not have a baby now she never will. She goes to Neil and asks him whether he would be prepared to provide some sperm so that she can have a baby. Neil agrees though he insists on having an antibody test 'just in case'. The antibody test is negative, so Neil and Sally proceed with the insemination.

But, unfortunately for both Sally and the baby, Neil is infected with the HIV virus. It's just that he has been so recently infected that antibodies have not had time to develop. Within five years Owen, Neil, Sally and the baby have died agonising deaths as the result of AIDS.

The two scenarios which I have just outlined are fictional. David, Sue, Bob, Owen, Neil and Sally are not real people. But the possibility that the HIV virus may be transmitted from individual to individual in the ways described is no fiction. A recent case reported from Belgium shows how far one person can spread the AIDS virus. The man in question, by all accounts exclusively heterosexual, made regular trips to Africa. In that time he had at least twelve sexual partners both in Africa and in Belgium. All of them were white, middle class, non-promiscuous, non-drug-using women whom he had met at parties. They all engaged in only vaginal intercourse with the man. The man himself is now dead — from AIDS. Nine of the twelve women have developed AIDS or ARC. One of the regular partners of one of the women has ARC.

What moral responsibilities do sexual partners have toward each other? What moral obligations (if any) does an individual who knows he is (or believes that he may be) infected with the HIV virus have to others in a situation of planned sexual interaction?

Since sexual transmission is one of the primary modes of transfer of the HIV virus this is clearly an important question. The details of how one answers this question will be determined by the view of ethics one takes. But since most ethical theories differ only with respect to the accounts they give of the nature of right and wrong and not in their evaluations of the rightness or wrongness of most forms of conduct, we can already expect that there will probably be a large amount of agreement on the question in which we are interested.

In this chapter, I will take two approaches to answering the question. The first is to look at the issue in terms of a conflict of rights. On this approach we need to be clear as to which rights, if any, a person who is HIV infected forfeits, and to whether those who are not infected gain any rights in societies where the AIDS phenomenon is a reality.

The second way of approaching the question is the utilitarian one, where we look at the issue not in terms of rights, but in terms of the consequences that will flow from adopting alternative courses of action. In this approach we need to look at the consequences of various possible interactions between persons, some of whom are HIV infected and some of whom are not. In this approach, how individuals should behave in these situations will be determined by which behaviours can be expected to give rise to the better consequences.

So let us return to David and Sue at that point in time when David has just become aware that he may be infected with the virus and so, if he goes on having unprotected sexual relations with Sue, he may be placing her at risk.

The rights theorist

What are the *prima facie* rights which come into conflict in this situation? David first. He has a *prima facie* right to express his sexuality in whatever way he sees fit, and to privacy with respect to his sexual preferences. He also has a *prima facie* right to know his antibody status. And then he even has a *prima facie* right *not* to know whether he is antibody positive (if that is what he would prefer!).

Now Sue. She has *prima facie* rights to life and health. More specifically she has a *prima facie* right not to be deceived by her husband about a matter with potentially serious consequences for her health.

On the rights approach our task is to impartially weigh the various rights of each party involved; that is, we must balance David's rights to privacy — with respect to both his sexual preferences and his antibody status — against Sue's rights to life, health and honesty from her husband in respect of these important matters.

Any impartial weighing of the rights involved in this case has

Sue's rights 'outweighing' David's, but still it seems that there are at least two ethically acceptable courses of action open to David at that point at which he becomes aware of the risks to himself and Sue of HIV infection. On the one hand he can tell Sue he is at risk and that she may be too. On the other he can have the antibody test.

Suppose David decides to take the test and the result is positive. What is he to do? The answer now is clear. He has a moral obligation to tell Sue his antibody status and let her decide whether she wants to continue to have sexual relations with him. Remember that the risks here are not trivial. It has been estimated that in a single year the risk of infection for a person engaging in regular sex with a partner who has the virus could be as high as 40 per cent. If either party has herpes or syphilitic sores, or if they engage in anal sex, the risk increases.

Any impartial weighing of the competing rights involved in the case of Sue and David will put Sue's right not to be exposed to risk of infection by the HIV virus ahead of David's rights to privacy with respect to sexual preferences and antibody status. In addition to this, a strong case can be made for the view that in entering into marriage an individual takes on particular duties toward his or her spouse. One of these particular duties will be a duty of care for the health of the spouse, a duty arising from the fact that the marital relationship is usually a sexual relationship.

Suppose now that the result of David's antibody test is negative rather than positive. David will undoubtedly be relieved to get this good news, but unfortunately unless he has had no extra-marital sexual contacts for the preceding three months he cannot assume on the basis of the result of this test that he is not infected with the HIV virus. He must wait another three months during which time he should not have sex with anyone who may be infected with the virus.

And he should not, this time for moral reasons, have sex with Sue during this three-month period — a course of action which could be expected to raise a number of domestic difficulties! How could David refrain from having sex with Sue for three months and *not* raise her suspicions? But let's suppose for the sake of the argument that he finds a way. David now goes and has a second antibody test and it too is negative. Finally, David has very good evidence that he is not infected with the HIV virus. And now he must make a choice. He may either continue with a genuinely monogomous relationship with Sue, or he can tell her about his other sexual relations, explain the risks, and let her make her own decision as to whether or not she is prepared to undertake the attendant risks.

Unfortunately, however, David's strategy of two antibody tests separated by a sex-free three months is open to an important moral objection. Remember our story. One day while she is out shopping Sue gives blood to the blood bank. Now suppose that David was indeed infected when he had that first antibody test, but the infection was too recent for the antibodies to have developed. Suppose further that Sue has already been infected. And suppose finally that Sue makes her blood donation during the three months between David's antibody tests. If Sue's blood is not detected to be antibody positive — and that is certainly possible since antibodies take some period of time to develop — it may infect others with HIV.

Unless David can be certain that Sue will not donate blood, he is not entitled to adopt the 'wait and see' strategy. If on the other hand there is some chance that Sue will donate blood, an impartial weighing of the rights of all those likely to be affected by David's decision shows that David has an obligation *right from the start* to tell Sue that he may be HIV infected so that she will not expose others to the risk of HIV infection by donating her blood. Any impartial weighing of the rights of all those likely to be affected by David's decision will put the rights to life and health of the anonymous recipient of a blood donation above David's right to privacy.

At first inspection it seemed that David had a choice with respect to telling Sue about his possible infection with the HIV virus — at least if his initial antibody test was negative. But, as we have seen, it would be only under very special circumstances that David would have such a choice — namely circumstances where he had very strong assurances that Sue would not unwittingly pass on the infection to others, through donated blood, pregnancy, extramarital sex or shared needles. The case of David and Sue shows just how easy it is for the HIV virus to be passed on. Individuals (like Sue) may be responsible for transmitting the virus to others because they have no idea that they themselves are infected.

The case of Neil and Owen raises the same set of ethical questions. The only difference between this case and the case of David and Sue is that Owen and Neil are living together in a stable homosexual relationship rather than as married heterosexuals. But with respect to the moral questions in which we are interested, this difference is unimportant. Like Sue and David, Owen and Neil have special responsibilities — notably responsibilities pertaining to the health of their partner — in virtue of the fact that they are living together in a long-term relationship. Any impartial weighing of the rights in question will accord greater weight to Neil's rights to life and health than to Owen's right to privacy about his drug use.

The utilitarian

We have seen how a rights theorist would handle our cases. Let's now look at what the utilitarian would say. David has just become aware that he may be infected with the HIV virus and that Sue therefore is also at risk. What is he to do?

The utilitarian will decide what David should do by looking at all the foreseeable consequences of the alternative possible actions open to him. He will take into account the fact that Sue may become infected with HIV and go on to develop AIDS or ARC. He will take into account the fact that Sue, unaware of the risk that she may be infected, may donate blood. He will take into account the fact that Sue may become pregnant and the child may be born infected with the virus. He will take into account the fact that David's revelation of his bisexuality may lead to Sue's throwing him out of the house, with all the psychological and financial ill-effects that this could be expected to produce. If Sue and David already have children the negative effects the breakup of the marriage may have on them will also be taken into account.

Having looked at all of these consequences, the utilitarian, like the rights theorist above, will decide that, in this case at least, David has an obligation to inform Sue that she is at risk of being infected with the HIV virus, since the consequences if Sue becomes infected and goes on to infect others are worse than the (admittedly also serious) consequences which may result if David tells Sue that he may be infected with HIV.

If David has an antibody test and the result is positive it is very clear that he has an obligation to inform Sue of the fact, for in this situation Sue is obviously at high risk of becoming infected herself.

What is less obvious (at least at first) is that a negative antibody test does not serve to justify the 'wait and see' strategy described above. Unfortunately, in situations like the one involving David and Sue, failure to appraise an individual that she (or he) is at risk may result in very bad consequences for other individuals. As we have seen, a woman who does not know she is at risk may donate blood and so place further individuals at risk. This is the fate that befell the unfortunate blood recipient Bob. And again, a woman of childbearing age infected without her knowledge may decide to have a child, whereas if she knew that she was infected she could avoid becoming pregnant.

It is important at this point to make it quite clear that I am not suggesting that there exists any *absolute* obligation for all persons at risk to have an HIV antibody test. There is no such obligation. Nor is there always an obligation to inform the spouse or lover that he/she may also be at risk. There may be the occasional case where this duty could be overridden — eg where the spouse or lover has a terminal disease such as cancer, will not live long, and would not donate blood anyway. But barring such unusual cases there will be a moral obligation on the person who is at risk of being HIV infected not to further expose to risk a non-consenting spouse or lover. And it is also wrong to fail to provide information that may prevent the spouse or lover being the cause of other individuals' suffering or death. This, morally speaking, is the bottom line.

CASUAL SEXUAL RELATIONSHIPS

We have so far been concerned with trying to establish the moral obligations that individuals living in long-term relationships — whether married or not — have toward each other. The time has now come to look at the somewhat more difficult question of what obligations casual sexual partners have toward each other. Short of long-term cohabitation there are many arrangements into which those in sexual relationships may choose to enter. Some married people choose to live in different houses or even different cities. Some people have extra-marital affairs that go on for many years. Indeed there is a whole continuum of arrangements between long-term relationships and one night stands, but for the sake of contrast I will concentrate on the one night stand.

Case 3

Jack and Sam meet in a gay bar. They have a few drinks together and return to Sam's apartment. It is clear that they are both considering the possibility of having sex.

Sam, who has recently had the antibody test, knows that he is antibody positive. What is he to do? If he tells Jack then Jack may no longer want to have sex with him. And, after all, Sam reasons, they have only known each other for a couple of hours. Sam feels he has no particular responsibility toward Jack. In fact they will probably never see each other again after this evening.

Case 4

Maureen and George meet at a conference. They spend a bit of time together, and as the week passes it becomes clear that they will probably have a fling.

After the conference dinner George invites Maureen back to his room for a drink. George has never had an antibody test, but since he has recently shared needles with other intravenous drug users, he knows that there is some chance that he could be infected with the HIV virus.

What is George to do? If he tells Maureen then she may no longer want to have sex with him, and he certainly has no special responsibilities toward her. They will probably never see each other again after this conference.

Is there an obligation to reveal one's positive antibody status to one's prospective casual sexual partner? And if one has not had the antibody test, but knows that there is some chance that one is infected, does one have an obligation to inform one's prospective partner of this fact?

Of course what one intends to do, or what it is reasonable to believe will happen, can make a serious difference. If the partners intend merely to engage in mutual masturbation, where there is essentially no risk if the skin that comes into contact with body fluids is not damaged, then there will be no obligation.

But suppose the couple plan to engage in either vaginal or anal intercourse, where the risks are high and very high respectively. In these cases the information in question is of the utmost relevance if an individual is to be able to make an informed decision about whether or not he or she still wishes to have sex. It is one thing to consent to have sex where there is a belief that there is no incipient danger to health and life that will flow from that action. It is quite another thing to consent believing such a danger to be present. Jack could well change his mind about this one night stand if Sam tells him that he (Sam) is antibody positive. And the fact that George could be infected with the HIV virus may well be information sufficient to dissuade Maureen from having sex with him.

Now let us continue with the story of George and Maureen. George and Maureen do not discuss the matter of HIV infection, but they do go on to have sex. A question which may now be raised is: what exactly did Maureen consent to when she agreed to have sex with George? Did she consent to HIV-free sex? Or did she consent to take the risk that George might be infected with the HIV virus?

There is a legal notion of consent, and its interpretation is a legally complex issue. But here we also have a moral issue. In a community where the dangers of HIV infection have been widely publicised and discussed, if an individual is not coerced into sex, is he or she *by that act* consenting to accept the risk that his or her partner is infected with the HIV virus? Maureen did not ask George whether he was at risk of being infected with the HIV virus. But should he have volunteered the information? And suppose that Maureen had asked George, would George then have been morally obliged to give her a truthful answer?

If we look at the question from the rights theorists' point of view then the rights we have to balance are George's rights to sex and to privacy about his drug use, and Maureen's rights to life, health and information about a matter with potentially serious consequences for her health. Any impartial balancing of these rights shows that George has an obligation to inform Maureen that he may well be infected with the HIV virus, or, rather, he has this obligation if he plans to continue with this sexual encounter. He could of course withdraw from the encounter rather than reveal information concerning his drug use — that is a perfectly acceptable course of action. But if he intends to continue he has a moral obligation to tell Maureen, and he has this obligation whether or not she asks him.

Now Sam and Jack. Again, Sam has a moral obligation to inform Jack that he is antibody positive. Jack's rights to life, health and to have information about a matter with serious consequences for his health clearly outweigh Sam's rights to sex and privacy about his antibody status on any impartial scale. Again, Sam has this obligation whether or not Jack asks him for the information.

The utilitarian will arrive at the same answers as the rights theorist in each of these cases. He will arrive at these answers because it is clear that the consequences of becoming infected with the HIV virus are so bad that they easily outweigh the bad effects of missing out on a sexual encounter, or even these bad effects *plus* the bad effects which could result from revealing that one is, or may be, infected with HIV.

The case for informing one's sexual partner when one knows one is, or believes one may be, infected with the HIV virus is very strong. But for those who, for one reason or another, may still harbour residual doubts, I have constructed some analogous cases with the aim of overcoming those doubts.

Case 5

Suppose I own a car hire business and all my cars are of one kind — Giottos. Suppose there has been a spate of accidents involving Giottos and it is suspected that there is some structural fault responsible. As yet no government action has been taken to prohibit anyone hiring out Giottos, but there has been lots of publicity, and there is a well-known theory that engines that are part of a particular run have been implicated in all the tragedies.

Suppose I am approached by a potential customer who I have reason to believe is also well informed about the spate of accidents, but who still wishes to hire one. I have one left in stock. Do I have a moral obligation to inform the customer that the car is equipped with an engine from the suspect run? More specifically, do I have an obligation to answer that customer truthfully if he or she asks me explicitly, and do I have an obligation to volunteer the information if he or she does not ask?

Case 6

Suppose I own a grocery store and stock just one very popular brand of baby food — Brand X. Suppose also that recently there have been a few 'strange' infant deaths and it is suspected that some cans of Brand X baby food with the 007 serial number are responsible, but as yet no government action has been taken to prohibit the sale of this brand with this serial number. However, there has been a lot of publicity of the theory implicating Brand X baby food.

Suppose I am approached by a customer whom I have no reason to suppose is uninformed about the infant deaths but she still wishes to buy some Brand X baby food. I have some in stock though it is all of the 007 serial number. Do I have an obligation to tell her that it has the suspect serial number? More specifically, do I have an obligation to answer her truthfully if she asks me explicitly, and do I have an obligation to volunteer the information if she does not ask?

One can look at each of these two cases in terms of a conflict of rights — on the one hand the customer's right to know about a substantive risk, on the other the vendor's right to make a profit. And the conflict is settled by an impartial weighing of these rights. Any impartial weighing in these two cases will show that the vendor has a moral obligation to inform the customer of the risk he or she will place himself or herself under whether or not a request for such information is made. Similarly if one takes the utilitarian approach and looks at consequences, one will reach the same conclusions. The very bad consequences which may involve loss of human life if the car is hired out or the baby food sold outweigh any good effects which may result from the vendor in question making an extra bit of profit.

In so far as the risks are of similar magnitude, and the consequences of similar severity, one's answers to these questions, and those raised with respect to the one night stand, should be consistent. Individuals may have a *prima facie* right to sex, but this right, like the storekeeper's right to sell goods, is not an absolute right that an individual has regardless of the consequences. I may have a right to sex but I don't have an absolute right to have sex with any particular person. The rapist cannot plead that he should be acquitted on the ground that he had a right to sex, and rape was the only way he could get any.

CONDOMS AND 'SAFE SEX'

The western world is currently engaged in an education program to promote 'safe sex'. Safe sex is something that we shall hear more about in Chapter 11. Safe sex may encompass many things — mutual masturbation is certainly very safe — but what is central to the safe sex program is the notion that using condoms whenever sexual interactions are likely to result in an exchange of body fluids will lower the risk of transmission of the HIV virus.

Does using condoms absolve an individual from informing his or her partner that he/she is (or may be) infected with the HIV virus?

The short answer to this question is *no*. Although condoms will reduce the risk of transmission of HIV, they do not necessarily eliminate that risk — the condom may tear or there may be spillage. And while this risk remains, a person is entitled to be in possession of information about the existence of the risk of HIV infection *before* deciding whether or not to have sexual relations with an infected person. After all, sex is (or at least should be) a purely voluntary activity. It's not like breathing which we must do if we are to continue to stay alive. I can choose to have sex with one person but not another. I can choose not to have sex with anyone. There is no obligation for me to have sex with anyone I don't want to have it with.

Using condoms will certainly reduce the risk of transmission of the HIV virus. But, again, if we impartially weigh the rights of the individuals involved, we see that this does not affect an individual's obligation to inform his or her partner if he or she has reason to believe that he or she is infected with HIV. Let us look again at the case of George and Maureen, this time assuming that they use a condom. Any impartial weighing of the relevant rights will accord precedence to Maureen's right not to be exposed to this (admittedly smaller) risk to her health. The utilitarian will reach the same conclusion. The consequences of infection with HIV are so very bad that even though using a condom means the risk of those consequences occurring is much lower, these consequences still outweigh any good consequences that could be expected to result from proceeding with the sexual interaction. Condoms have their uses, one of which is to lower the probability of transmission of HIV. But using condoms cannot absolve an individual from the responsibility of informing his sexual partner that he may be infected with the HIV virus and therefore could transmit the virus.

When the consequences of a course of action are very serious and the risk that these consequences will be actualised non-negligible, the ethical conclusion one is forced toward, using a utilitarian framework, a theory of rights and duties or indeed, say, application of the Golden Rule, is one in which the relevant information is supplied whether (or not) a request for such information is made. If we apply the Golden Rule we see that it is clearly in the best interests of an antibody negative individual that he or she not be exposed to HIV. When the HIV infected individual 'puts himself or herself in the position of the non-infected individual' it will become clear to that individual that he or she has a duty to inform his or her prospective sexual partners about that HIV infection.

ADDITIONAL READING

Mann, J. 'The Global Strategy for AIDS Prevention and Control' Geneva: World Health Organisation, May 5, 1987

QUESTIONS

1 Do some individuals have particular responsibilities for others in virtue of special relationships, for example, parent to child, wife to husband, lover to lover?

2 How would a utilitarian answer question 1?

3 How would a rights theorist answer question 1?

4 Do sexual partners have responsibilities toward each other? Has AIDS changed these responsibilities?

5 'I'm infected with the AIDS virus because someone else chose to behave irresponsibly. So why should I bother about protecting anyone else from catching it.' What do you think about this position?

6 'So long as I use condoms I'm being responsible.' Suppose the person who says this is antibody positive. Do you agree with him or her? In answering, look at a range of sexual activities — petting, masturbation, vaginal sex, anal sex.

7 'If I tell people I'm antibody positive then they mightn't want to sleep with me. So I'm not going to tell anyone. I'll use condoms instead. After all, that makes sex safe, doesn't it?'
What do you think about this position?
Does it make a difference if the people are
  (i)   married?
  (ii) living together?
  (iii) involved in a one-night-stand?

4 FROM ETHICS TO DISCRIMINATORY POLICIES

In this chapter my project will be one of determining what criteria must be met before the state is entitled to intervene and discriminate against some classes of individuals. When do we discriminate? Well, we discriminate when we do not allow one individual to do 'the very same thing' as another. The South African government, for example, discriminates against blacks when it prohibits them from buying houses in 'white only' areas. The white man may buy a house in such an area, but the black man is prohibited from doing 'the very same thing'.

In our day-to-day speech the word 'discriminate' carries various negative connotations. To admit that an action is discriminatory is already to acknowledge that the action is morally wrong. There is another use of 'discrimination' according to which one discriminates when one treats different individuals differently, but where there is no presumption or connotation that the discriminatory treatment is morally wrong.

JUSTIFIED DISCRIMINATION

Within our community it is accepted that, whether they want to or not, individuals with tuberculosis may be isolated from the rest of the community until they are cured. If we were to treat tuberculosis carriers in the same way as non-carriers — that is, if we were to let them continue to live freely within the community — it would be unfair to the other members of the community. We could have a tuberculosis epidemic and many people would die. Someone might argue here that it is unfair to isolate individuals with tuberculosis from the rest of the community because it is not their fault that they have the disease. But while isolating individuals with tuberculosis may have some unpleasant consequences for those so isolated, the consequences would be worse if we did not take measures to protect other individuals from catching the disease.

Another example of defensible discrimination is limiting the right to vote to people above a certain age. In Australia those below the age of eighteen do not have the right to vote. Individuals below the age of eighteen are discriminated against in this respect But this piece of discrimination seems justified because children generally are not well informed about political and economic matters. Moreover, allowing young children to vote would facilitate a situation where parents were effectively given control of additional votes. So, all in all, discrimination against children in this matter may well be justified.

More generally, if the consequences of non-discrimination are sufficiently bad then discrimination may be justified. Put another way, discrimination may on occasion be justified as a means of achieving a particular desirable end. The health of the community is a major priority and this justifies the discriminatory practice of quarantining those with tuberculosis. Achieving a fair and responsible vote is another major priority which justifies the discriminatory practice of excluding those under eighteen from voting.

But how are we to determine whether the consequences of non-discrimination qualify as 'sufficiently bad'? Discriminating against some individuals, that is, treating them differently from others, will often have undesirable effects for those discriminated against. Therefore the benefits or end that a discriminatory policy aims to produce must at the very least be sufficient to justify the means employed to produce it.

UNJUSTIFIED DISCRIMINATION

It would be wrong to refuse to employ a person *just* because that person happens to be a woman, or black, or homosexual. If the job is one of designing bridges, whether the person happens to be female, black, homosexual or a white Anglo-Saxon Protestant male is clearly irrelevant. What is relevant is whether the individual has appropriate training and the necessary work experience. To the extent that job applicants have equivalent qualifications and experience they should be treated equally.

Suppose we have a situation where a number of individuals apply for a job that involves designing bridges. The candidate best qualified for this job in terms of both qualifications and experience is a woman — Mary. But the person doing the hiring — George — believes this kind of work is unsuitable for a woman. So he hires another candidate — Fred.

Like the government that requires that individuals infected with tuberculosis be non-voluntarily isolated in order to prevent the spread of that disease, George too has an aim. His aim in effecting his discriminatory policy is to keep women out of civil engineering, since George believes that a woman's place is in the home looking after children.

But the aim of preventing the spread of tuberculosis is defensible in a way in which keeping women out of civil engineering is not. A policy which isolates individuals infected with the tuberculosis bacillus will keep more people healthy than would be the case in the absence of such a policy. Put another way, the rights of healthy individuals to continue to be healthy outweigh the rights to freedom of movement of those infected with the tuberculosis bacillus. An impartial consideration of the effects that implementing such a policy would have, and comparison with the effects that could result if such a policy were not implemented, will lead to the implementation of such a policy.

But how can we *know* that we have given impartial consideration to the effects of implementing, as opposed to not implementing, a given policy? The contemporary American philosopher John Rawls argues that a principle is fair, or impartial, if it is one that we would all agree to if we were to make our decision from behind a veil of ignorance. Rawls' veil of ignorance is a veil which obscures from us all the particular aspects of our lives which may consciously or unconsciously cause us to vote for particular social arrangements because they benefit us as individuals. The kind of thing Rawls' wants to rule out is a situation where, say, a man votes for sexist employment practices because this will perhaps make it easier for him to get good jobs and a high income.

> The idea... is to set up a fair procedure so that any principles agreed to will be just... Somehow we must nullify the effects of specific contingencies which put men at odds and tempt them to exploit social

and natural circumstances to their own advantage. Now in order to do this I assume that the parties are situated behind a veil of ignorance. They do not know how the various alternatives will effect their own particular case and they are obliged to evaluate principles solely on the basis of general considerations... First of all, no one knows his place in society, his class position or social status... (Rawls, 1972: 136)

Now let us return to George and Mary. George's discrimination against Mary cannot be given the justification that can be given to the practice of discriminating against those infected with the tuberculosis bacillus since George has *not* impartially weighed all the rights of all the parties involved. Mary's rights to employment and to be treated fairly — to name just two — have been accorded insufficient weight. If Mary had been a man then George would have given her the job. He would have accorded her rights to employment and to be treated fairly their proper weight — that is, the same weight he has accorded to Fred's rights to these things. Put another way, if George had been forced to make his decision without knowing the sex of the various applicants then he would have chosen differently. He would have chosen Mary.

In situations where the consequences of an act of discrimination are bad, and these negative consequences do not appear to be counterbalanced by any overriding positive ones, we will have reason to suspect that the rights of the individuals involved have not been weighed impartially. Alternatively, if an act of discrimination results in far better consequences than would have occurred in the absence of that discrimination we will have reason to feel confident that the rights of those involved have been weighed impartially.

EVALUATING THE JUSTIFIABILITY OF DISCRIMINATION

Because of the negative effects of discriminatory policies, discrimination is only justified in those circumstances where the consequences of non-discrimination are sufficiently bad. How then are we to determine whether the consequences of non-discrimination qualify as 'sufficiently bad'? In other words, does the end indeed justify the means?

We all agree that it is reasonable to prohibit those with very bad eyesight from driving motor vehicles on public highways. Similarly, most of us agree that it is reasonable to isolate insane individuals who pose a danger to others until such time as they are no longer dangerous. But what about less obvious cases? What about the law that prohibits the sale of alcohol to individuals below the legal drinking age? And what about the law that prohibits cinemas from admitting those below the age of eighteen to R-rated movies?

Is it justifiable to exclude minors from activities like drinking in pubs or viewing R-rated movies merely because they have not attained the age of eighteen? Given that alcohol consumed to excess is bad for the health of the individual and may in some circumstances develop into an addiction, there is a *prima facie* case for the interference in question. However, whether actual interference — discrimination — is justified depends on the answers we get to questions like the following:

1 How bad is the harm?
2 How likely is it that the harm will actually eventuate?
3 Can those responsible for the harm be accurately targeted?
4 How bad are the effects of the discrimination itself ?
5 How confident are we about our answers to the above questions?

Before going on to discuss whether discrimintion against people infected with the AIDS virus is justifed it will be useful to look in more detail at each of these important questions.

1. How bad must the harm be before discrimination is justified?

The simple answer to this question is that the consequences must be bad *enough*. For example, slightly unpleasant consequences should not do, but life threatening ones may. An example of this kind of difference is the difference between having typhoid and having a very mild cold. There is a high probability that an individual who contracts typhoid will die, and so discrimination here in the form of non-voluntary quarantining is justified on the ground that others should not be exposed to the risk of contracting the virus in question. In the case of a very mild cold, however, discrimination in the form of non-voluntary quarantining is not justified because having a mild cold for a few days is not sufficiently bad, and the consequences of such a quarantine are arguably worse.

Of course, it is really more complicated than this. For example, how widespread the consequences will be is also relevant. Mildly bad consequences for many members of a population may well be enough to justify discrimination, while mildly bad consequences for a small sub-population would not be.

2. How probable must the harm be before the discrimination is justified?

It is not required that the population *has already experienced* the consequences, or that it be certain that it would unless the discrimination is enforced. What is required is that it can be predicted with an appropriate level of probability that the consequences would occur unless there is discrimination. With a new disease that resembled the bubonic plague it would not be necessary to wait until half the population of the country were dead before a discriminatory policy in the form of a non-voluntary quarantine would be justified. To wait until 50 per cent of the population had perished would clearly be silly. There will also be circumstances in which some pre-emptive discriminatory action will be justified. When the first astronauts returned from the moon they were quarantined for a period of time in order to ensure that they had not brought back to Earth any potentially lethal organisms. It's not that the scientists had evidence that they were indeed carrying any such organisms, but then neither was there any evidence that they were not. The costs associated with isolating the astronauts were small, whereas the potential benefits of this action, if indeed they turned out to be carrying dangerous organisms, were very high. And so isolating the astronauts was justified.

In all cases of proposed discriminatory action a careful balancing of the expected consequences that would flow from the implementation of a discriminatory policy and those that would flow from the non-implementation of that policy will be necessary in order to determine whether the discriminatory policy is justified.

3. Can those responsible for the harm be accurately targeted?

If we were to allow those who do not have good eyesight unrestricted access to the roads in motor vehicles this would have bad consequences for the population as a whole. In short, there would be many accidents. But those who do not have good eyesight divide into two groups — those who wear glasses and those who do not. Those who neither have good eyesight nor wear glasses will be even more likely to produce carnage on the roads, while those who do not have good eyesight but who *do* wear glasses will be only infinitesimally more likely to cause accidents than the individual with normal eyesight.

In this case we should only discriminate against drivers who do not have good eyesight *and* do not wear glasses. It would be wrong to ban all those who have bad eyesight from the roads regardless of whether or not they wear glasses. More generally, there is a moral requirement that we discriminate against only those who *actually* pose a threat to the community. To do otherwise is wrong.

In the not too distant past an issue of this kind was vigorously debated in the context of the exclusion of women from certain occupations. Some argued that quotas limiting the number of women entering courses like medicine and engineering were justified because women generally had less aptitude and interest in these subjects than did men. But even supposing that women generally did have less aptitude and interest in these areas, it was unjust to impose quotas to limit their entry. The women who did not do as well as their male counterparts in entrance examinations could already be excluded on that basis.

If there are a limited number of places for students to learn a particular profession then selection according to academic merit is a justifiable mode of selection. Selection on the basis of sex is not, for it is far too crude a method of selection. Even if we accept that males generally have better visual-spatial skills than females — and there is evidence that this is so (Maccoby, E. and Jacklin, C., 1974) — there are many females who have better visual-spatial skills than many males. It is unjust to exclude women as a group when we already possess the means — namely examinations or tests — whereby we can look at the individual's ability to perform certain relevant tasks.

4. Will the discrimination itself produce bad effects and do these bad effects outweigh the good?

Discriminatory policies that aim to produce positive results may 'backfire' and produce a situation worse than that which the policy aimed to alleviate. Suppose for the sake of argument that reliable university tests had shown that children from families with annual incomes below $10 000 were highly likely to have head lice. Head lice spread very quickly through populations of school-aged children, and being infested with lice is not a good thing. Suppose now that a plan were proposed whereby children from families with annual incomes below $10 000 would all be regularly deloused during school hours.

It is reasonable to expect that such a plan would bring about a radical reduction in the number of cases of head lice among school-aged children, but it does not require much imagination to see that such a policy would result in those unfortunate children who were regularly deloused suffering all sorts of ill-effects as a result of this policy. Other children could be expected to laugh at them, ostracise them and generally victimise them. In short, the negative social consequences of such a policy could well outweigh the positive. Schools could be made lice-free by such a policy, but the cost would be too high. The bad effects of this discriminatory policy would outweigh the good.

Furthermore, the process of ascertaining which individuals are the members of the class to be discriminated against may have such bad effects that it would be preferable to abandon that particular discriminatory policy. Doubtless many more drug pushers could be apprehended if the police were given wider powers to search people, vehicles and premises. But would we want to give the police such wide ranging powers? After all, if they were given them, individuals could be guaranteed very little privacy, and this bad effect may well outweigh the good effects which would certainly flow from the apprehension of more drug pushers.

5. How confident can we be about our answers to the above?

While science has done much to give us a greater understanding of the nature of the physical world, scientists are certainly not infallible. Even if we use the best information and theories available it is still possible to be wrong when making predictions concerning the future.

Beginning with Malthus in the eighteenth century, there have been those who have predicted that human populations would grow so quickly that over-population and starvation would soon be endemic on the planet Earth. While there is serious over-population and starvation in countries like India and Pakistan, other countries have not experienced similar effects. In the West, for example, contraception and safe abortion have brought about significant reductions in birth rates, and over-population is no longer perceived as a threat. Even in countries where contraceptives are not readily available, green revolutions have occurred and population growth has been contained. In China, for example, families are permitted to have only one child. If a woman becomes pregnant after bearing her one child she can either have an abortion or cope with the many problems raised by the fact that this child has virtually no legal rights. Not surprisingly the Chinese policy has been effective in keeping down the birth rate. When Malthus made his predictions he did not foresee the green revolutions nor the advent of effective contraceptives and safe abortion. He was wrong about what the future held, but his mistakes were reasonable given the information he then had about agriculture, populations and population growth.

What is true of Malthus' prediction could also be true of many current scientific forecasts. Take the contemporary concern with the state of the ionosphere. Scientists are predicting that chemical wastes now being pumped into the atmosphere will result in a destruction of the ionosphere which will lead to the planet becoming significantly hotter. The seas will rise, islands will sink, the weather will become less predictable, there will be more cyclones and skin cancers. But then maybe science will discover a way to replenish the ionosphere so that none of the predicted bad effects will occur.

Even the best of scientific predictions have not proved infallible. The fact that not all scientific predictions have been verified does not mean that we should take no notice of what science has to tell us about the future. Since we have no direct access to what the future holds, the best we can hope to do is to work out what seems the most likely outcome, given the information we have, and then act on this evaluation. This is the course of action that can be expected overall to generate the most positive consequences. To refuse to base policies on the best evidence available will only serve to increase the probability of bad consequences occurring.

Another problem arises from the fact that many predictions are couched in the language of probability rather than necessity. This raises the difficult question of what level of probability of the bad consequences occurring is required before discrimination becomes justified. Obviously this cannot be determined independently of the nature of the consequences. But what is clear is that a mere *possibility* of bad consequences is not sufficient. If we take life threatening consequences for an entire population, we would tolerate only a very small probability before discriminating (unless the discrimination itself carried with it a higher probability of equally bad consequences), but for mildly unpleasant consequences for a sub-population, the probability tolerable would obviously be higher.

There are also questions concerning the accuracy of probability estimates. At election time in particular it is clear that there is little consensus among commentators about which polls are truly indicative of the preferences of the electorate. Two factors that are important, however, are that the sample is of sufficient size and is 'representative' of the population being surveyed.

An election forecast based on a survey of three individuals would be based upon a sample that was far too small. On the other hand, a forecast made on the basis of a survey of individuals leaving a Liberal Party meeting would be non-representative. Similarly, it would be inappropriate to exclude all girls from woodwork classes on the basis that not one girl in the two metropolitan schools surveyed wished to do woodwork. And it would be irrational to conclude that 50 per cent of eggs are rotten on the basis of once having bought a dozen, six of which were rotten .

Finally there is the problem of what we are to do with respect to cases where no research has been done to determine the probability of bad consequences occurring in a particular kind of situation. This is an issue that has often been raised in connection with AIDS. Some parents, for example, have argued that since no scientific studies have yet been done to determine the probability of HIV being transmitted by a human bite, it is not acceptable to allow children infected with that virus to attend school.

While it is certainly true that there has been no study to determine a numerical value for the probability of transmission of the

HIV virus through human bites, we do have a lot of more general information about the nature of this virus, and this information supports the view that the probability in question will be extremely low. Many cases in which no numerical value can be assigned to a risk will be like this — that is, we will still have some reasonably good idea of the magnitude of the risk involved even though an exact numerical value cannot be assigned to it.

AIDS AND DISCRIMINATION

It is now time to turn to the question of whether some form of discrimination against those infected with HIV is justified. Let us briefly review the medical picture of this virus, and of those who have been infected with it.

The most serious cases of infection are those where the individuals have full-blown AIDS. Such individuals typically have severe, life-threatening, 'opportunistic' infections, such as certain kinds of pneumonia and cancer, due to deficiencies in their immune systems. Less serious cases of HIV infection are those with AIDS Related Complex or ARC. These individuals are not in immediate danger of losing their lives, but are in very poor health and great discomfort. There are also individuals who have had a confirmed antibody positive test result for HIV, but have no symptoms (that is, they are quite healthy). And finally there are individuals infected with the HIV virus but who have not been tested or have not shown up as antibody positive when tested, either because the test has failed or because there has been insufficient time for antibodies to develop.

All those who are infected with HIV are potentially contagious to others. So do we have a case for discriminating against all those infected with the virus? Certainly the consequences of being infected with HIV are sufficiently bad. One will suffer a very painful death if one goes on to develop AIDS. One's quality of life suffers considerably if one (merely) goes on to develop ARC. The chance that these serious consequences will eventuate if individuals go on living their lives as if AIDS did not exist is significantly high. And finally, since extensive research underlies these estimates it is rational to act upon them.

Discrimination against individuals simply on the ground that they are infected with HIV fails miserably, however, with respect to both the moral and practical requirements discussed above. In the first place it is impossible to tell just by looking at a person whether or not he or she is infected with the virus. Indeed the person himself may be unaware he or she is infected with the virus. Take for example Sue, who is married to Dennis. From time to time Dennis uses IV drugs and has shared infected needles. Sue is infected with the virus, but since Dennis has never told her about his drug use, and she has no symptoms, she has no idea that she is.

The moral objection to discriminating against all those infected with HIV (if indeed we were able to distinguish all of them just by looking) is that many of those so infected constitute no danger to others. Remember that AIDS is transmitted through close personal contact, that is, through sex and blood. You can't get AIDS through sharing bathrooms or tearooms and you can't get it by breathing the air infected individuals have breathed. If someone is infected but never again enters into the kinds of close personal contact by which the virus is spread he or she poses no threat to anyone.

Discriminating against individuals on the basis of their being infected with HIV is not acceptable on either pragmatic or moral grounds. But there is of course an obvious solution for getting around the practical problem: regular testing for everyone in the community.

The big advantage of this approach is that we would then have very accurate information on the size of the AIDS problem and the rate at which it is growing. But there are also weighty reasons against regular universal testing. The first is that it would be astronomically expensive. Admittedly the expense could be curtailed if the tests were less frequent, and even infrequent tests would be useful to epidemiologists. The less regular the tests, however, the more inaccurate the information would be since there would always be individuals who had become antibody positive since the last test.

Maybe we could live with these inaccuracies. But what about the consequences for those individuals who test positive? It is not easy to live with the news that you are antibody positive when there is a high probability that you will go on to develop AIDS or ARC. But more importantly there is the problem of the link which exists between AIDS and homosexuality. Homosexuals already suffer discrimination within our society. Individuals with AIDS who are homosexual may suffer even greater discrimination, and heterosexual men infected with the virus may be discriminated against because it is assumed they are homosexual. A similar story can be told with respect to intravenous drug use and so it is plausible to argue that the good consequences of universal testing would be outweighed by these bad consequences. Indeed many advisory services counsel individuals against being tested, for these very reasons.

One way of reducing the monetary costs of testing would be to compulsorily test only those belonging to high risk groups. But here again there are both pragmatic and moral objections. It is impossible to tell simply by looking who belongs to a high-risk group. Most intravenous drug users do not go around advertising the fact, nor do many homosexuals and bisexuals. The wives of bisexuals frequently are not aware of their husbands' bisexuality. Any attempt to find out whether individuals belong to high risk categories would, of necessity, be highly intrusive and unacceptable as a gross invasion of the privacy of the individual. Such attempts would themselves lead to very bad consequences.

There is again the fact that in most ordinary social interactions an HIV infected person is no threat to the health of others. Take again our individual who knows he is infected and thereafter refrains from those close personal interactions that may lead to the spread of the virus. He is no threat to anyone, and there is no reason to discriminate against him. Public Service Board decisions not to discriminate against antibody positive individuals accord with this view. They are justified by the fact that the probability of the HIV virus being transmitted from one individual to another in normal interactions in an office is, after all, infinitesimal.

Before leaving the question of compulsory testing is there anything more which can be said in favour of it? Some have argued that individuals belonging to high risk groups should be tested, because a positive test result will lead them to modify their behaviour. If they are not tested, the argument goes, they will continue to behave in risky ways and the virus will be passed on to more people. David Pennington, who until recently was head of the AIDS Task Force, is one who holds this view.

The evidence on whether a positive test result leads to favourable modifications in behaviour is inconclusive. Research done in Holland and Canada has shown that people who tested antibody positive were reducing the number of their sexual partners more radically than those who tested negative. But would these individuals have modified their behaviour without the test? After all, most of them would have had reason to believe themselves to be at risk, even without the test. Other surveys done in Baltimore, Chicago and France found that changes in the sexual behaviour of homosexuals were unrelated to antibody test results, although there was a significant positive correlation between information about AIDS and safer sexual practices.

Further research may lead to a better understanding of how knowledge of antibody status affects subsequent behaviour. In the meantime, however, a policy of anything other than voluntary testing seems unjustified, though, as we will see later, individuals who choose not to be tested will have extra obligations toward others. Investigations aimed at seeking out all those belonging to risk groups would be unjustifiably intrusive, and in all probability ineffective. It is also implausible that the majority of those at risk would actually come forward voluntarily.

AIDS is a frightening disease and it would be much better for all of us if it did not exist. Given that it does exist we are fortunate that its mode of transmission is not like that of various influenza viruses. One can catch the flu merely by breathing in air that contains infected droplets of moisture that other individuals have breathed out. But you cannot get AIDS that way. To get AIDS there has to be an exchange of body fluids, and now that blood banks are screened, for all practical purposes that means through sex and the sharing of infected needles.

Unlike breathing, which is an involuntary action, individuals usually have a choice as to whether or not they have sex. An individual who is infected with HIV virus is usually in the position of being able to choose to behave responsibly: he or she can refrain from sexual activity, or appraise his or her prospective partners of the potential risks. With respect to drugs the situation is a bit more tricky, for here there is the difficult question of whether the situations in which the virus is transferred are likely to be ones where individuals have a real choice with respect to behaving responsibly. But generally the kinds of considerations we have been looking at push us in the following direction. We should only discriminate in those cases where it is reasonable to believe that there is a high risk that a person is both infected with HIV and will not behave responsibly. Discrimination against those in high risk groups, or even against those who have confirmed antibody positive test results, should not be automatic.

It would of course be desirable not to discriminate (socially or legally) against any of those who are HIV infected or have a high probability of being so infected. But this view rests on the presumption that such persons will accept certain responsibilities and obligations in their interactions with others. And of course if there is failure to be responsible, or if it is reasonable to believe that some persons will not behave responsibly, then there will be a strong case for discriminatory treatment.

We earlier discussed the difficulty in deciding whether a person is HIV infected, or at high risk of being so infected. It might be thought these concerns are minor compared to those required in making a judgement concerning a person's propensity to act responsibly. But then this judgement is one we commonly make in a whole range of personal and public situations, and so there is no reason to think we cannot make it here.

CASES WHERE DISCRIMINATION MAY BE JUSTIFIED

To behave in a morally responsible manner is to behave in a way that minimises the probability that bad consequences will be brought about. It is obvious that a necessary condition for an individual to be able to behave responsibly is that he (or she) have the capacity to act freely, that is, to choose, and that there is no compulsion, mental abnormality or mental incapacity that makes this impossible.

Discrimination is justified in just those cases where it is reasonable to believe that an individual (or group of individuals) has been, or is at high risk of having been, infected with HIV and cannot be relied upon to behave responsibly. Let us now consider four such cases to see why discriminatory treatment may be justified in the circumstances outlined.

The HIV infected blood donor

All states and territories within Australia now have legislation requiring blood donors to sign declarations that they do not belong to any of the risk groups for HIV infection. Those making false declarations are subject to legal penalties of varying degree. In NSW it is $5000, one year's imprisonment, or both. In Victoria a person can be fined 50 penalty units, imprisoned for two years or both. In Queensland imprisonment can be for a term of up to two years and one can be fined up to $10 000.

Such legislation is discriminatory against those who know themselves to belong to groups at high risk for HIV infection since, unlike those not belonging to high risk groups, these individuals are excluded from donating blood. But while this policy may be discriminatory it would be recognised by virtually everyone as discrimination which has the strongest possible justification.

The HIV infected psychotic

Certain kinds of psychosis render an agent not responsible for his or her actions, or at least not responsible while he or she is undergoing a psychotic episode. If we have reason to believe a psychotic has been infected with HIV, and the probable behaviour of this person places others at significant risk of becoming infected, restriction of his or her freedom of interaction may be justified.

The HIV infected IV drug user

Injecting intravenous drugs with a dirty needle is one of the more probable ways of becoming HIV infected. Intravenous drug users who are HIV infected may place other IV drug users at risk of infection if they share needles or syringes with them. And they may also place their sexual partners at risk.

Because of their drug dependence some intravenous drug users may not be able to be relied upon to behave in a morally responsible manner with respect to this matter. Others may simply choose not to be responsible and therefore discriminatory action which restricts the freedom of interaction of intravenous drug users may in some circumstances be justified.

HIV infected children

Children infected with HIV are another group for whom discriminatory policies may be justified. Since older children can to some extent be relied upon to behave responsibly, it is very young children who, because of their lack of mental and moral development, potentially constitute the most pressing problem. It may therefore be argued that their right to non-discriminatory treatment is lost.

The HIV infected person who is sexually irresponsible

We have already discussed what constitutes sexually responsible behaviour for the HIV infected individual. But what if an individual *chooses* to behave in a sexually irresponsible manner?

This case differs from those involving psychotics, IV drug users and children in that all of the latter (for one reason or another) may be incapable of behaving in a morally responsible manner in situations likely to lead to transmission of HIV. The sexually irresponsible individual, on the other hand, is a danger to the health of others because he or she *chooses* to behave irresponsibly.

Take for example a promiscuous individual who has had many sexual partners, or has had sexual contact with people who are HIV infected. If this individual continues to have sexual relations with others whom he or she does not appraise of the facts of his or her sexual history that individual is behaving in a manner that may warrant discriminatory treatment. In assessing the individual's moral culpability one must tackle the difficult question of whether that individual can be said to *know* of his or her HIV infection in the absence of an antibody positive test result. But certainly if a person has had the test and been informed of a positive result that person does know that he or she is infected. A discriminatory policy can be targeted without difficulty to this latter class of individuals.

There are cases where HIV infected individuals cannot be relied upon to behave responsibly. If this lack of reliability stems from a mental inability or incapacity, different measures will be called for than those that are appropriate when dealing with individuals who are capable of behaving responsibly but *will not*. What particular measures are appropriate will be determined by the detailed nature of the situation in question and I shall continue with a more detailed discussion of these matters in Chapters 5–8.

ADDITIONAL READING

Maccoby, E. and Jacklin, C. *The Psychology of Sex Differences* Stanford: Stanford University Press, 1974
Rachels, J. (ed.) *Moral Problems* New York: Harper and Row, 1976
Rawls, J. *A Theory of Justice* Oxford: Oxford University Press, 1972
Singer, P. *Practical Ethics* Cambridge: Cambridge University Press, 1979

QUESTIONS

1 What is discrimination?
2 When is discrimination not justified?
  Answer with examples.
3 When is discrimination justified?
  Answer with examples.
4 What is the moral difference between discrimination against individuals
  (i) on the basis that they are black, and
  (ii) on the basis that they are insane and hence dangerous?
5 What is wrong with the suggestion that all people infected with the HIV virus should be quarantined? Consider both moral and practical difficulties. Do you find the difficulties trivial or serious?
6 Some people have suggested that all those belonging to high-risk AIDS groups should be tested for antibodies.
  (i) What are the arguments in favour of this proposal?
  (ii) What are the arguments against it?

(iii) Does it make a difference if the testing is
   (a) voluntary?
   (b) non-voluntary?
7 Should people who know they are infected with the HIV virus be prevented from having sex with others?
8 Should people infected with the HIV virus be legally required to inform their sexual partners of this fact?
9 What should be done about young children who are carriers of the virus?
10 What should be done with those who are infected with the HIV virus and who deliberately expose others to risk?

5   What Is the Law For?

TED: The problem with the law today is that it's just too soft. You can rape and murder and be out in ten years. Why the hell should these people get off so lightly? No wonder there is no respect for law and order any more.

ANNE: But what is the point of keeping people in prison if there is no reason to suppose they will commit any more crimes? And it's not fair to keep someone in prison after he has paid his debt to society.

TED: But that is just the point I am making, Anne. He hasn't paid his debt to society. He hasn't paid his debt to anyone. A criminal rapes or kills in the most brutal fashion, and all that happens is that *society pays* to have him kept in reasonable circumstances for a few years. Where is the justice in that?

ANNE: But there is no point in keeping him in prison when he is no longer a danger to others. The law is meant to be concerned with justice, not vengeance. Isn't it better for him, his family and for society generally that he returns to become a useful member of it? Then we don't have to pay for his keep or for his family's either.

TED: That is just where I disagree with you, Anne. The punishment should fit the crime. That's what law is all about, or at least it should be.

ANNE: But you can't allow prisoners to be tortured or sexually abused just because that is what they did to their victims. We live in a civilised sociey and that would be barbaric.

TED: Well I agree, but that just means you have to keep them locked up for a lot longer or perhaps even execute them. Even that isn't equivalent to what they have done, but at least it's more in the right direction. Anyway it's not just what that criminal would be likely to do. If penalities were harsher there would be less crime. People would be put off becoming criminals.

ANNE: I know everyone says that, but I think studies have been done — in Sweden or somewhere like that — which show that harsher punishments do not deter people from committing violent crimes.

TED: Maybe that is so, Anne. I personally doubt it, but maybe you're right. But my original point remains. It's unfair to dole out feeble punishments for violent crimes, and it's bad for society. Imagine how the family of the victim feels. I'm surprised there are not more individuals who take the law into their own hands to get some real justice.

ANNE: Ted, you've already admitted that the law could not rape or torture criminals, so what is all this talk about 'real justice'? The law isn't about exacting vengeance for private individuals. The purpose of the law is to do what is best for society as a whole.

TED: Like how?

SARAH: Well, to make life in communities possible. That means there have to be rules and it's pointless having rules if there are not sanctions to back up those rules. If individuals knew they could break the law any time they felt like it and not be punished there would be total chaos.

TED: But Anne has already argued that experiments have shown that punishment does not deter people from committing crimes.

SARAH: In my opinion it is really beside the point whether people are deterred or not. What is important is that it is made clear that society will not tolerate certain kinds of behaviour.

TED: You and I, Sarah, both agree that society should step in and punish individuals who disobey the rules. So why don't you think that sentences should be more severe?

SARAH: Well, maybe they should, Ted. But I think it's important to see that the questions are quite distinct. The question of how heavy the sentence should be is quite distinct from the question of what is the purpose of the criminal law. Anyway, that is how it seems to me.

ANNE: But not to me. I think the questions are closely connected. The purpose of the criminal law is to help make things as good as they can be for the community. Punishment harms the people who are being punished, and so punishment is only justified to the extent it prevents even greater harm.

TED: I don't agree with you either, Sarah. Criminals should be punished because they have done wrong. And because the things they have done are horrible moral wrongs, not just trivial ones, they deserve serious punishments.

Under the Australian federal system, as in the United States of America, criminal law is primarily a state matter. The Commonwealth (or Federal) Government is empowered to make laws on certain specified matters including customs, defence, taxation, currency and social security. But with respect to most other matters each state has its own laws.

Within Australian jurisdictions the criminal law is founded upon the traditional principles and practices of English criminal justice, that is, it derives from the common law of England. However during the early years of this century Queensland, Western Australia and Tasmania codified their criminal laws, and so the statutes which make up each of the codes came to replace that part of the common law upon which they were based as the primary point of legal reference. New South Wales, Victoria and South Australia have not similarly codified their criminal laws. But over the years these three states have introduced large numbers of statutes regulating matters once covered only by common law. What is the difference between statute law and common law? The major difference is that statute laws are laws written down and passed by act of parliament, while with common law systems, some laws can be traced back only to judicial precedents but not to any legislation.

Very much more could be said about our criminal laws and the workings of the criminal justice systems in Australia. In this chapter, however, I will be concerned with a more general question, namely, what is the fundamental purpose of the criminal law?

There are three distinct philosophical conceptions of the purpose and nature of criminal justice, which are usually found combined in the views of most people: criminal justice as a method of crime prevention, criminal justice as moral criticism, and criminal justice as social criticism.

CRIMINAL JUSTICE AS A METHOD OF CRIME PREVENTION

According to this view the purpose of criminal justice is to reduce (and hopefully eradicate) crime. The aim is not only to correct the inclinations of the convicted criminal, but also the correction of the inclinations of those who have not yet committed crimes. According to this view, punishment of criminals will both correct and deter.

The main objection to this view is that there is good evidence to believe that a large number of serious crimes are one-off affairs, and unlikely to be repeated by their perpetrators even in the absence of any punishment. This is because most violent crimes are committed against victims the assailant knows, and with whom some relationship already exists. In addition to this there is evidence that punishing a particular individual for a crime does little to deter others from committing similar crimes. Punishing Fred for murder does little to deter Bill or Barry from committing murders.

A second objection is that the system of criminal justice we actually have is particularly ill-suited to the task of crime prevention. To prevent crime it would obviously be best to identify those with dangerous proclivities *before* they commit their crimes. This fact, that our system of criminal justice is not well suited to the task of crime prevention, may be seen as indicative of radical inadequacies in our system of criminal justice or, alternatively, the inadequacy of this conception of criminal justice. However, a scheme under which those with dangerous tendencies, but who had not yet committed crimes, were tracked down and given treatment to eliminate those tendencies differs so radically from the system of

CRIMINAL JUSTICE AS MORAL CRITICISM

According to this view, crime is morally wrong and the punishment of crime is justified by this fact. What is correct about this view is that those crimes of violence — murder, rape, assault — which stand at the core of any criminal code are certainly moral wrongs. When these crimes are committed moral wrongs are also perpetrated. Crimes like tax evasion may also be seen as morally wrong, though for a different reason — they place an unfair burden upon others. Criminal acts may also be seen as morally wrong by virtue of the fact that they weaken the rules of the society by allowing the criminal an unfair advantage over those others who exercise restraint and obey the rules.

There are good reasons for rejecting the view that it is the moral wrongness of an act that jusitifies its punishment by the law. In the first place there are acts that are morally wrong but are not crimes, for example, betrayals of confidence, breaking promises and certain kinds of lying. There are good reasons why the law does not intervene in such cases. The cost of intervening in these cases outweighs the benefits: there would be difficulties in enforcing such laws, and the liberty and privacy of individuals would be interfered with in a way not justified by the harmfulness of the acts in question.

Most crimes may indeed be moral wrongs but it is not their moral wrongess alone that makes them crimes.

CRIMINAL JUSTICE AS SOCIAL CRITICISM

According to this view the criminal law forges the limits of socially tolerable conduct and prohibits acts outside those limits. The criminal law establishes rules of conduct whose observance allows us to enjoy life in society, and ensures these laws are taken seriously by making their violation punishable. According to this view, those acts which pose a threat to the existence of a society should be crimes. This view allows for the separation of law and morality. Some moral wrongs, for example murder, are also crimes. Other moral wrongs, for example lying and breaking promises, are not.

The criminal law is primarily concerned with controlling the harm that any individual may do unto others. However, the law is not usually interested in penalising individuals who do harm unintentionally or accidentally. Nor does it punish individuals for being inadequate or unworthy people. The law concerns itself only with *acts* of individuals. Before the individual may be punished for an act, it must be established that he or she has acted *culpably*.

Human beings may be harmed in many ways. Great harm is done to individuals by earthquake, bushfire, volcano and similar acts of God. Other harms are caused by human beings, for example road accidents. The criminal law is only interested in humanly instigated harms, but certainly not all of them. In order to establish the guilt of a defendant in the criminal court it is necessary to establish *mens rea* (guilty mind). A successful plea of insanity, for example, is sufficient to establish the non-existence of *mens rea*, and so an insane individual who kills another cannot be found guilty of murder.

Some humanly instigated harms are not criminal acts. Similarly there are cases where no harm in fact occurs but where there is culpable conduct and thus criminal liability. Three interesting subclasses of the above category are unsuccessful attempts, reckless acts, and negligent acts .

Attempts

There must be a death before there can be a homicide. If the bullet misses then the most serious charge that can be laid is attempted murder. But various attempts are in themselves crimes. These attempts are all attempts that, had they succeeded, would have resulted in crimes of a very serious nature — death, serious bodily injury, rape, or robbery. Trivial offences usually do not have attempt liability.

Recklessness

Conduct in which there is indifference to the inherent dangers associated with the activity in question is reckless conduct. A driver who speeds at 180 kph through a built-up area may be charged with reckless driving even though no actual harm may result. In this case, the driving itself is seen by the law as culpable conduct, because it is conduct that *very easily* could have resulted in grave harm to others.

Negligence

Some activities in which we engage have certain risks associated with them, and it is incumbent upon those engaging in such activitites to do so with safety. Failure to take *sufficient* care when engaging in an intrinsically risky activity, where that activity brings about harm to others, is negligence. Suppose a crane is being used to unload containers from a ship. A small and unobtrusive sign warns pedestrians of the risk of walking in the area under the crane. Fred does not see the sign, and he walks into the area and is killed by a container which accidently falls. Fred's death was caused negligently, for those operating the crane were engaging in an intrinsically dangerous activity and they failed to take adequate precautions to prevent harm occurring to passers by.

There is no attempt liability in the case of either negligence or recklessness. This is because behaviour which may correctly be described as a (failed) attempt at negligence or a (failed) attempt at recklessness is behaviour too far removed, causally, from the harm that, in other circumstances, may have ensued. For example, a drunken individual who gets into his car but before pulling out from the kerb is detained by the police may strictly speaking be described as attempting to perform a reckless act (ie attempting to drive while intoxicated). But since the driver never leaves the curb, he or she at no time poses an *actual* threat to the safety of anyone, and is therefore *not* liable to prosecution.

THE COSTS OF CRIMINALISATION

Criminalisation of *any* activity carries with it some costs. Judges and policemen must be paid, and individuals charged with criminal offences are frequently removed from the work force while they await trial. An individual found guilty of a serious offence is then typically removed from the workforce for an extended period of time. Not only does this individual become a burden on the taxpayer, but his family may be left without means of support and they are then likely to also become a burden. Additionally, criminal trials cost a lot of money.

There are many crimes committed in Australia that usually go unpunished. For example, dozens of televisions, videos and stereos are stolen every day, and if one is the victim of such a crime one's chances of recovering one's goods or of seeing the thieves brought to justice are minute. Many members of the community are critical of the inadequacy of our law enforcement institutions. Thus the question must be asked: would a radical expansion of the police force and/or stiffer penalities for individuals convicted of these crimes do much toward reducing the level of such crime? And, would the costs of that expansion be justified by the increase in the rate of conviction? Certainly it would be better if one's property were more secure, but this security has a price. Every dollar which is used to pay for this security is a dollar not available for education, health care or any of the large number of other worthwhile government projects.

In addition to these obvious monetary costs there are also important non-monetary ones. If we give liberty its classic definition as 'the absence of legal coercion' then the citizen's zone of liberty is defined by the law. According to this definition liberty is not just an absence of any kind of constraint, but rather the absence of particular prohibiting rules backed by the threat of punishment. If there is no law to prohibit bigamy then an individual is free to have as many spouses as he or she wishes. In our society an individual is not free to have more than one spouse, and is therefore less free *in this respect* than a man living in Saudi Arabia. More generally, the point is that criminalisation of behaviour means that the liberty of individual citizens is reduced.

Most, if not all, liberal writers have endorsed a 'presumption in favour of liberty'. What this means is that *ceteris paribus* (other things being equal) a citizen should be left free to make his or her own choices. There are good reasons for endorsing this 'presumption in favour of liberty'. To begin with, a person deprived of a liberty suffers a genuine loss. Secondly, liberty encourages creativity in its broadest sense. An individual who is free to choose can be expected to develop his or her decision-making skills. In general, such a society will cope better with unforeseen changes.

But while, *ceteris paribus*, a citizen should be free to make his or her own choices, there clearly are many cases where other things are not equal. In *On Liberty* John Stuart Mill argues that interference with an individual's liberty is only justified in order to prevent harm to others. Subsequent writers have both elaborated upon and diverged from this view, but the fact remains that the criminalisation of an activity results in a loss of liberty for at least some members of the community. Since liberty is a good, this loss must constitute a cost associated with criminalisation.

There is also a less obvious but no less important cost which may accompany the criminalisation of an activity. This cost can best be described as a loss of respect for the authority of law. When will this cost be incurred? To answer this question it is necessary to digress momentarily in order to describe the legal background against which a new law is introduced.

Suppose we have a criminal code which prohibits a small number of violent crimes and nothing more. Suppose further that there are effective law enforcement agencies — that is, there is a high probability that someone who breaks the law will be caught, found guilty and punished — and that the penalties for these crimes are substantial. In this society virtually all those who commit crimes are caught and punished severely.

The criminal code just described is *effective*, and will be seen as such by the population. We could expect that in this community there will be respect for the authority of law. Given this legal background we may reasonably expect that a new law which is not similarly enforceable (for whatever reason) will not substantively diminish that community's respect for the authority of law. Indeed, at least initially, we might expect the new law to be respected and obeyed, because the other laws have been and continue to be successfully enforced, but we cannot go on indefinitely adding unenforceable laws to a criminal code without at some point there being a substantial diminution in respect for the rule of law. Any existing criminal code already contains laws which are difficult to enforce, and so to criminalise some activity where there is little probability of enforcing the new law carries with it the cost that there will be a general lessening of respect for the rule of law.

It should also be noted here that there are frequently alternatives to criminalisation, alternatives which may well achieve a similar result. One non-penal method of controlling anti-social behaviour is via taxation. Cigarette smoking is not only dangerous to those individuals engaging in it. It also affects the health of others who inhale the exhaled smoke. Since much of our medical care is paid for through taxation, smokers who suffer emphysema, lung cancer or any of a number of other bronchial complaints caused or at least exacerbated by smoking are placing an extra burden on the non-smoking portion of the taxpaying community. The taxing of cigarettes is one way of both controlling and paying the costs of an activity which imposes costs upon others.

Other non-penal methods of controlling anti-social behaviour include job dismissal from public agencies, suspension of welfare payments, loss of custody of children, or withdrawal of professional certification. Suspension of welfare payments has actually been used in Australia. Earlier this century a man became ineligible to receive an old-age pension if he had deserted his wife and failed to provide for her and their children!

While not technically interferences with the liberty of the individual, these sanctions are clearly punitive, and they bring with them the additional cost that the individual sanctioned does not have the rights and protections accorded by the criminal law to an individual accused of committing a crime.

AIDS AND THE CRIMINAL LAW

As we have already seen, there are five main groups of HIV infected individuals who pose a threat to the health of others. They are:

1 The sexually irresponsible
2 The IV drug user who shares syringes
3 Certain psychotics
4 Some infants and small children
5 Some blood donors

As argued in Chapter 4, discrimination against those infected with HIV in certain circumstances may be justified. Those circumstances, in brief, are ones where individuals cannot be relied upon to behave responsibly and thus pose a threat to the health of the community. Our aim now is one of determining whether any of the kinds of behaviour which may lead to the transmission of HIV are appropriate objects of concern for the criminal law.

Crimes of violence, such as murder, rape and assault, stand at the core of any criminal code. All these crimes involve significant harm to others. The culpable transmission of the HIV virus to an 'innocent' individual, or acts involving significant risk of such transmission, must be seen at least *prima facie* as at that core too. After all, to contract either AIDS or ARC is to suffer a significant harm.

According to *any* of the three conceptions of criminal justice outlined above, prevention of the culpable transmission of AIDS to innocent individuals is *prima facie* a proper concern of the criminal law. According to the first conception (criminal justice as a method of crime prevention), the purpose of the criminal law is to reduce (or maybe even eradicate) crime. Thus, the use of the criminal law to prevent innocent individuals from being infected with AIDS seems appropriate, or at least as appropriate as it is to the prevention of other crimes of violence. According to the second conception (criminal justice as moral criticism), the transmission of AIDS to an 'innocent' individual, or reckless behaviour that could easily result in such transmission, is behaviour that may rightfully be punished under a criminal code, since such behaviour, which has a significant probability of causing serious harm to an innocent individual, is certainly morally wrong. Finally, according to the third conception (criminal justice as social criticism), legislation criminalising activities which may lead to the contraction of AIDS by innocent individuals is again at least *prima facie* appropriate since if these activities place innocent individuals at risk of suffering serious harm, then a case can be made that the behaviour in question lies beyond socially tolerable limits.

There have been, and still are, long disputes concerning the merits and demerits of these three competing conceptions of criminal justice. What I have done is sketch these views, and indicate what I consider to be the crucial inadequacies of two of them. It is my view that the third view (ie that criminal justice is a form of social criticism) is correct. However, due to the nature of the issue under investigation, most of what I will now say will be true whichever view of the nature of criminal justice one holds. The three conceptions of criminal justice all reach similar conclusions with respect to the justice of punishing crimes like murder, rape and assault. The transmission of the HIV virus or reckless conduct likely to lead to its transmission poses a threat of harm to others where that harm is of a magnitude similar to that caused by assault or rape. So we might therefore have *expected* that, independently of the view of the nature of criminal justice one happens to hold, one will come to the conclusion that it is justifiable to criminalise culpable conduct with the potential to lead to the transmission of the HIV virus.

As we noted earlier, the criminal law is not in business to penalise individuals who do harm unintentionally or accidentally. It will therefore be an unsuitable tool for dealing with those HIV infected individuals who are either mentally ill, immature or incapacitated, and have behaved in a manner which has (or is likely to have) transmitted the HIV virus to another individual.

But what of those individuals who are capable of behaving responsibly but who *choose* not to? Again, we have already noted that the criminal law is concerned only with *acts* of individuals, so there can be no criminal sanctions imposed upon an individual in the absence of his or her committing a culpable act. Criminal sanctions cannot be imposed just because it is probable that an individual will commit some such act.

The criminal law may only be used in cases where an individual has *already committed* a culpable act. With respect to the matter of the transmission of HIV, that class of acts which meets all of the above constraints is a subclass of the class of acts of sane, adult, HIV infected individuals. Individuals who know they are infected with the HIV virus and still behave in a sexually reckless manner appear to be appropriate objects of the criminal law.

A *prima facie* case certainly exists for criminalising those sexual behaviours of sane, adult, HIV infected individuals which may lead to the infection of other, innocent individuals. The question we must now examine is whether this case is more than a *prima facie* one.

ADDITIONAL READING

Gross, H. *A Theory of Criminal Justice* Oxford: Oxford University Press, 1979

Lyons, D. *Ethics and the Rule of Law* Cambridge: Cambridge University Press, 1984

Mill, J. S. 'On Liberty' in *Utilitarianism, Liberty, Representative Government* New York: Everyman, 1968

NSW Public Health (Proclaimed Diseases) Amendment Act 1983, No. 183

Queensland Health Act Amendment Act (No. 2) 1984, No. 103

Sallmann, P. and Willis, J. *Criminal Justice in Australia* Melbourne: Oxford University Press, 1984

QUESTIONS

1 Make a list of actions that are morally wrong but against which it would be inappropriate to have laws.
2 When (if ever) should the law enforce morality?
3 What do you think of the popular view that the primary purpose of the law is to deter people from committing crimes? Do you think that some laws are more likely than others to act as deterrents? Name the laws and give reasons why you think they do, or do not, deter.
4 Do you think it would be better if the law were changed so that a violent person could be detained before he or she actually killed someone? What would be the advantages of such a system? What would be the disadvantages?
5 Do you think the law should be changed so that a person who has committed a violent crime can be brainwashed to make him non-violent (as in Kubrick's movie *A Clockwork Orange*)? What are the arguments for this proposal? What are the arguments against it?
6 What do you think of our laws concerning marijuana? Compare them to those regulating the use of alcohol. Is it reasonable to be so much 'harder' on those who use marijuana than on those who use alcohol?

6 AIDS AND THE CRIMINAL LAW

The American states of Idaho and Florida have made it a crime for persons infected with the HIV virus to knowingly expose others to the risk of infection. In Britain the Public Health (Control of Diseases) Act 1984 allows for patients believed to have AIDS to be compulsorily examined and for AIDS patients to be removed to and detained within hospitals. The Soviet Union has recently announced that an individual infected with HIV who continues to have sexual relations is liable to imprisonment of up to five years, and if the virus is actually transmitted then that person may be imprisoned for eight years. In Australia, New South Wales has made it illegal for an individual infected with HIV to have sexual relations with another without first appraising him or her of the fact that he or she is so infected. Queensland has made it an offence for a person to infect another with the HIV virus unless the persons are married or living in a de facto relationship *and* the uninfected person has agreed in advance to take upon himself or herself the risk involved. These latter laws in Queensland and NSW are very different. In NSW an HIV infected individual who informs his or her sexual partner of the fact that he or she is infected has discharged his or her legal duty, and cannot be held responsible if that person later becomes infected. In Queensland, on the other hand, there may be cases where an individual who infects another can be fined, jailed or both, even though he or she has informed his or her partner in advance of the risks involved, *and that partner has agreed to proceed regardless of the risks*. Later in this chapter I shall discuss the legal situation in other states, but for now let us look at the law as it applies in NSW.

The NSW Public Health (Proclaimed Diseases) Amendment Act of 1985 curtails the sexual activities of persons infected with the HIV virus in the following manner:

50N. (1) In this section, 'sexual intercourse' means —
    (a) sexual connection occasioned by the introduction

> into the vagina, anus or mouth of any person of any part of the penis of another person; or
> (b) cunnilingus.
> (2) For the purposes of this section, a person shall not, only because of age, be presumed incapable of having sexual intercourse.
> (3) Any person who knows he or she has a proclaimed disease shall not have sexual intercourse with another person unless, before the sexual intercourse takes place, the other person
> (a) has been informed of the risk of contracting a proclaimed disease from that person; and
> (b) has voluntarily agreed to accept that risk.
> Penalty: $5000.

Of course there would be a significant problem in establishing that an individual *knew* that he or she was infected with HIV if there were not also legislation requiring doctors to notify some central authority of the occurrence of HIV antibody positive test results. In NSW there is such legislation, for the Proclaimed Diseases Amendment Act of 1985 also requires medical practitioners and pathology laboratories to notify the secretary of the Department of Health of all HIV antibody positive results. This notification must be done in code to ensure confidentiality — doctors are prohibited from using a patient's name and address when requesting a pathology test or notifying the secretary. Such a system will allow for the retrieval of the name of an HIV antibody positive person in certain circumstances. In brief, if the Chief Health Officer of the Department of Health has reasonable grounds for believing that ascertaining the identity of the person is necessary for the purpose of safeguarding public health, he may apply to the District Court for an order requiring the doctor to release the name of the antibody positive individual.

The NSW AIDS legislation has been widely criticised as counter-productive if its aim is that of stopping the 'spread of HIV. Some have argued that the criminalisation of sexual behaviours likely to lead to the transmission of HIV will result in more (rather than fewer) people becoming infected with the virus, since if an individual who has *not* been tested for HIV infection is safe from legal repercussions this may discourage him or her from being tested. Others have argued that even a coded notification system of antibody positive test results will reduce the number of individuals being tested, since the existence of a mechanism for tracing the name of an individual could lead to discrimination against him or her. The fact that AIDS is a 'minorities' disease (the two highest risk groups are male homosexuals and intravenous drug users) has made the gay community nervous about the possible uses to which such a list of HIV infected individuals could be put. It was only as recently as 1984 that homosexual acts in private between consenting adults were decriminalised in NSW, and homosexuals still suffer the effects of being a minority in a predominantly 'macho' culture. The process of assimilation into the community at large has not been helped by the AIDS crisis.

The general difficulty raised by those opposed to the legal measures taken in NSW in response to the AIDS crisis is that notification of antibody positive test results will discourage people from being tested, and the criminalising of sexual behaviours will even further discourage them. But let us look more closely at the problem. Being or not being tested is, in itself, unimportant. It is through sexual activity (and sharing syringes) that HIV infected individuals spread the HIV virus. Morally responsible individuals who believe they may be at risk of being antibody positive will behave in a sexually responsible manner *whether or not* they have been tested. Presumably, some HIV infected individuals will be so irresponsible that they will behave in a reckless manner even after they have had the test and know themselves to be antibody positive. But the class of individuals of interest to us here is neither of the above. Rather it is that class the members of which will not have the test and so will behave irresponsibly, but *would* have behaved responsibly if they had had it.

Immediately following the NSW AIDS legislation, there was a dramatic reduction in the number of individuals presenting themselves for HIV antibody testing. But then the numbers rose again. While this does not show that some individuals who would have been tested if there were no legislation have now been dissuaded from doing so, it does show that the community at large has not been dissuaded from being tested by the new laws.

While public attention has focused on the worry that the NSW AIDS legislation will discourage individuals from being tested and so (arguably) lead to an increase in the sexual transmission of HIV, there are other costs associated with the prohibition in question. In the first place, if vigorous attempts are made to enforce the law, then the existing law enforcement facilities must be either extended or spread more thinly. Second, it is clear that the liberty of at least some individuals is diminished — those who have tested antibody positive are no longer free to engage in sexual intercourse without telling their partners their antibody status. And finally, since these kinds of laws, for obvious reasons, will be difficult to enforce, it is arguable that such laws will contribute to a general loss of respect for the rule of law. The last mentioned difficulty is not by itself sufficient cause to allow an undesirable practice to flourish unchecked. As the law stands it is frequently difficult to obtain a conviction of rape, but then such a difficulty is rightly seen to count for little when weighed against the gravity of the offence in question. All the same, this cost remains one to be kept in mind and accorded an appropriate weight.

In short, these are the costs associated with the NSW AIDS legislation. But are there any benefits? Do the benefits outweigh the costs? With a view to answering these questions I shall look at a number of hypothetical cases to see what legal difference the NSW AIDS legislation has made.

Case 1

Mrs McX has lately grown suspicious of her husband, Mr McX. He is staying out late and offers no explanation. At first Mrs McX suspects he has acquired a mistress, but then she discovers a stack of homosexual pornography in the woodshed. Her suspicions grow. Finally, she confronts him with these suspicions but he refuses to discuss the subject. Mrs McX has been having sexual relations with McX until the very recent past. She has read about AIDS. She is convinced that McX is bisexual and that she may have caught HIV. She goes to have a blood test. It is positive. She goes to the police.

Before NSW AIDS legislation

There is nothing the police would do for Mrs McX, since they would not recognise her infection as being the result of any crime. Mrs McX may have been infected with HIV but she has no symptoms and does not appear to be suffering in any way — it is certainly not obvious that she has suffered any harm. Mr McX has done nothing against any law by continuing to have sexual relations with her, even if he knows that he is HIV infected and may therefore infect her too. If the police are particularly sympathetic to Mrs McX and consult a lawyer to see if there is any possible ground for apprehending McX they will discover that there is no general principle that makes the transmission of a communicable disease a criminal act.

Suppose now that Mrs McX goes on to develop AIDS or ARC. Can she now do anything? Well, once again she would be faced by the practical problem that the police would not recognise her illness as being the result of any crime for the reasons outlined above. And again there would be the difficulty that there is no general principle that makes the transmission of communicable disease a criminal act. But now at least it is clear that she is suffering some actual harm and so it is *technically possible* that a criminal action could be brought.

Let us suppose that Mrs McX dies from AIDS. And let us further suppose that a criminal action against McX is brought, charging him with the murder of his wife. Is there any chance of this action succeeding?

It would appear that *at the very least* Mr McX has acted negligently in failing to inform his wife that he is antibody positive, while continuing to have sexual relations with her. Since Mr McX will have also been aware of the non-negligible probability that a serious harm may be suffered by his wife in consequence of his actions, and since he owes her some duty of care (in virtue of the fact that it is foreseeable that his act could result in serious consequences for her), it seems that he should be liable.

But can more be established? Can *mens rea* be established in this instance? Is it plausible to argue that McX intended to kill his wife?

Establishing mens rea

One possible defence that McX's lawyer may now employ is to argue that his client did not intend to kill his wife. On the contrary, McX's intention was the completely innocent one of (say) wishing to have a good time, and so it would be inappropriate to find him guilty.

If McX's lawyer argues that his client's intention was merely that of securing for himself a good time, and therefore he cannot be guilty of murder, he will be using the kind of defence employed in the famous case of Hyam. The facts of that case, as presented at the final appeal to the House of Lords, were as follows (the *appellant* is the person making the appeal, in this case Hyam, the woman on trial):

> For some time the appellant had been J's mistress but their relationship ceased in consequence of the appellant suffering from some gynaecological trouble. Thereafter the appellant became suspicious of J's relationship with a Mrs B; she made attempts to break up that relationship by writing anonymous letters. Eventually one night she drove to the house where Mrs B was living with her son and two daughters, and set fire to it. She did nothing to alert the occupants of the house to the danger she had put them in, or the fire brigade, but drove back to her home some five miles away. As a result of the fire Mrs B's two daughters were killed. The appellant was charged with their murder. She admitted that she realised that what she had done was very dangerous to anyone living in the house but said that she did not intend to cause death or grievous bodily harm; she was jealous of Mrs B whom she believed was about to marry J, and her motive in starting the fire was to frighten Mrs B into leaving the neighbourhood. (*All England Law Reports*, 1974: Vol 2, 41)

At the trial of Hyam the judge directed the jury that if they were satisfied that when Hyam set fire to the house she knew it was highly probable that this would result in death or serious injury to those within then it would be true to say that she intended to kill or seriously injure those within, and her claim that she only intended to frighten Mrs Booth was irrelevant. The trial judge wrote down the following passage and gave it to the jurors to take with them to the jury room .

The prosecution must prove, beyond all reasonable doubt, that the accused intended to (kill or) do serious bodily harm to Mrs Booth, the mother of the deceased girls. If you are satisfied that when the accused set fire to the house she knew that it was highly probable that this would cause (death or) serious bodily harm then the prosecution will have established the necessary intent. It matters not if her motive was, as she says, to frighten Mrs Booth. (*All England Law Reports* 1974: Vol 2, 44)

Hyam was found guilty of murder by the jury. Her defence appealed to the Court of Appeal. The appeal was dismissed, but the Court of Appeal gave Hyam leave to appeal to the House of Lords on the ground that the decision involved a point of law of general public importance, namely the question:

Is malice aforethought in the crime of murder established by proof beyond reasonable doubt that when doing the act that lead to the death of another the accused knew that it was highly probable that the act would result in death or serious bodily harm?

The House of Lords answered this question in the affirmative. They argued that in order to establish the *mens rea* for murder it was sufficient to prove that when the accused performed the relevant action he (or she) knew that it was probable that this action would result in grievous bodily harm to another. In consequence of this, Hyam's appeal was dismissed. She was guilty of murder because the jury had been satisfied that when she set fire to the house she realised it was highly probable that someone within could suffer serious bodily harm as a result of her action.

This ruling is of obvious relevance to the case of transmission of HIV we are now discussing. It means that *mens rea* can be established even in the absence of a particular conscious intention of the form 'I'll give her AIDS!' With respect to the case of McX all that needs to be established is that when McX had sex with Mrs McX he knew that it was probable that his action would result in grievous bodily harm to her.

When is an event probable?

Is it right to claim that it was probable that Mrs McX would suffer serious consequences as a result of McX's action? When does something that is possible become probable? If the probability that an event will occur is 6:10 is this event probable? What about a probability of 1:10, 1:20, 1:50? If I hold a loaded gun with five empty chambers at the temple of another, pull the trigger and kill him, would (should) I be found innocent of murder on the ground that there was a (mere) 1:6 chance that he would be killed? We assume not. But is this judgement based solely on the magnitude of the probability involved, or does the fact that a person who holds a loaded gun to the head is already acting recklessly (and therefore culpably) influence our estimation?

Someone who engages in heterosexual intercourse (when not infected with HIV) will usually not be acting recklessly. The probability of HIV being transmitted through any particular act of heterosexual intercourse is very much lower than 1:6. If, as seems correct, it is a good deal less than 1:50, then it is unclear what the law would (should) say with respect to a casual sexual encounter — the prototypical 'one night stand'.

The case of McX is not one where there is a single isolated sexual encounter. Numerous acts of intercourse over a significant period of time increase the probability of Mrs McX becoming infected. If McX continues to have sexual intercourse with his wife knowing that he is infected with the HIV virus, then after some interval of time it will become plausible to contend that it is *probable* that Mrs McX has become HIV infected.

The problem of evidence

Another serious difficulty faced by the prosecution in attempting to convict McX concerns evidence. The world we live in is one where we do not have perfect access to information. Additionally, our criminal code is one in which innocence is assumed until guilt has been established *beyond reasonable doubt*. To begin with, there is the problem of establishing whether or not McX informed his wife about his antibody positive state. Suppose Mrs McX claims on her death bed that McX had not informed her and suppse McX claims that he did in fact inform her and that she agreed to undertake the risk.

There is of course the question of whether or not Mrs McX

contracted AIDS as a *causal* consequence of her sexual relationship with McX. Suppose Mrs McX is not a faithful wife, and that she has had a number of other sexual contacts in the period of time during which she became infected. If one of these other contacts is infected with HIV or if any contact cannot be located then it will be open to McX to argue that Mrs McX may well have contracted AIDS from that person rather than from him.

To establish beyond reasonable doubt that an individual contracted AIDS as a result of his/her sexual contact with some other specific individual will, in many circumstances, be fraught with difficulty. It may not be impossible, but it certainly will not be easy. Furthermore the whole question of the admissibility of the previous sexual history of the victim of a crime raises problems. Recently there has been much debate about the admissibility of the woman's sexual history in a rape trial. Whatever the rights or wrongs of the admission of such evidence, it seems that it would be very difficult for a defendant to establish that someone other than himself or herself may have transmitted the AIDS virus to the victim if that victim's sexual history is inadmissible evidence.

After NSW AIDS legislation

The police are now in a position to do something for Mrs McX since under the Public Health (Proclaimed Diseases) Amendment Act of 1985 it is an offence for an individual who knows he or she is infected with HIV to expose his or her sexual partner to the risk of infection without first appraising that person of the risk. The police will recognise that Mrs McX's HIV infection may be the result of a crime.

What can the police do? They can approach the Director of Public Health who may obtain an order from the District Court for Mr McX's doctor to release information concerning McX's antibody status, if such information exists. Let us suppose McX has indeed been tested and that the result of the test was positive. If it can be established to the satisfaction of the court that McX knew that he was antibody positive, and that he had intercourse with Mrs McX without appraising her of this fact, then it is possible that he will be convicted.

Suppose now, contrary to the original story, that McX has not had an HIV antibody test. In this case it is unlikely that any charge would be brought. However the Director of Public Health may instruct McX to be tested, and McX is legally obliged to follow this instruction. This may provide little consolation for Mrs McX, but at least it ensures that there can be no repetition of a scenario in which McX is invulnerable to the law.

An individual who has had an HIV antibody test is, from a legal point of view, more vulnerable than one who has not had the test, for usually there will be no problem in establishing that such a person *knows* himself or herself to be HIV infected. As mentioned earlier, this is a concern that has been voiced by many in connection with the NSW AIDS legislation, and it is usual for such critics to go on to argue that we therefore would be better off without the legislation. So let us for a moment consider another possibility. Suppose this legislation were framed so that it was no longer requisite that the individual *knows* that he or she is antibody positive (in the sense that it is not necessary that he or she have had an antibody test and be aware that the result is positive). Suppose rather that *having reason to believe* that there is a high probability that he or she is HIV infected is all that is required. If this were the case then it would be possible to establish culpability even in the absence of a positive test result. Mr McX would not be invulnerable simply because he had not been tested.

Any attempt to modify the law in this way will generate more problems than it solves. In the first place there is the question of what constitutes sufficient reason for believing that there is a high probability that an individual is infected. Would being a member of a high risk group be sufficient to establish potential culpability? Suppose McX had been an active bisexual for many years. Would this *of itself* establish his potential culpability?

Any change to the law in the direction proposed above has the potential to be overtly discriminatory with respect to certain minorities in a way in which the actual legislation is not. The actual legislation is framed in a way which is completely neutral with respect to sexual preference and with respect to whether an individual is an intravenous drug user. *Any* person who knows he or she is HIV infected has an obligation to inform his or her prospective sexual partners of the fact. Although the Public Health (Proclaimed Diseases) Amendment Act 1985 may allow some of the sexually irresponsible to escape the law, it is to be preferred to an alternative of the kind just outlined, which could well prove to be overtly discriminatory against homosexuals, bisexuals, and intravenous drug users.

What if Mrs McX develops AIDS?

Suppose finally, as we did before, that Mrs McX goes on to develop AIDS and dies. Does the Public Health (Proclaimed Diseases) Amendment Act 1985 make it more likely that McX may be found guilty of murder? The short answer to this question is that probably it does not, but if it does, then it does so only slightly. McX behaves in a legally culpable manner when he becomes aware that he is HIV infected but continues to have sexual relations with Mrs McX while not appraising her of the risk. His behaviour is reckless in the same way that the behaviour of the motorist speeding through the shopping centre is reckless. But while it will be easy to establish that this motorist is *causally* responsible for the deaths of any pedestrians he or she knocks down and kills, it will not be similarly easy to establish that Mrs McX has been infected with HIV *by McX* . And if the McXs have only had sporadic sexual encounters (something that is not improbable if McX is bisexual) it could well prove difficult to establish that McX's behaviour made it probable that Mrs McX would become infected.

Case 2

Mrs McY has lately become suspicious of her husband, Mr McY. He frequently returns home in the early hours, and often appears out of touch with reality. At first Mrs McY suspects he has acquired a mistress, but one day she discovers a used hypodermic syringe in the glovebox. Her suspicions grow. Finally she confronts him with these suspicions but McY refuses to discuss the subject. Mrs McY has been having sexual relations with him until very recently. She has read about AIDS. She is convinced that McY is an IV drug user, and that she may have been exposed to the HIV virus. She has a blood test. It is positive. She goes to the police.

As far as the law is concerned this case is in all essentials the same as Case 1. *How* McY acquired the HIV virus is unimportant.

Case 3

Dr P has been treating the McGs for a number of years. McG has aroused his suspicions, and Dr P believes McG to be something other than what he presents himself as — a middle class pillar of society. McG has come in from time to time with complaints not usually suffered by pillars of society. One day McG asks Dr P to arrange for him to have the HIV antibody test. The result is positive. Later that month Mrs McG comes to see Dr P, not about the result of the antibody test, but for a rather severe cold. As she is leaving she says to Dr P, 'I hope the next time I'm in, it will be for a pregnancy test. We've been trying for a number of months, you know!'

Before the NSW AIDS legislation

Dr P can do nothing.

After the NSW AIDS legislation

Dr P can lodge a complaint with the police. As with any complaint, the police will conduct an investigation. This will include establishing that McG has been antibody tested, and is indeed antibody positive. It will also include interviewing Mrs McG to determine whether or not McG has appraised her of his antibody status. If McG has informed her, the investigation will be terminated. But if Mrs McG claims that McG has not informed her, criminal proceedings could ensue. Obviously Mrs McG's attitude will now be of vital importance in determining whether or not a conviction is obtained. If she chooses to protect her husband it is unlikely that he will be found guilty.

Case 4

Dr J has been treating the McWs for a number of years. McW has aroused his suspicions. Dr J believes McW to be something other than what he presents himself as — a middle class pillar of society. McW has come in from time to time with complaints not usually suffered by pillars of society. This time it is suspected anal herpes and gonorrhoea. Dr J suggests to McW that maybe he could also do a test for the HIV virus. McW refuses, claiming that there is no way he wants such a thing 'on the record'. Later that month Mrs McW comes to see Dr J, for a rather bad cold. As she is leaving she says to Dr J, 'I hope the next time I see you it will be for a pregnancy test. We've been trying for a number of months, you know!'

Before the NSW AIDS legislation

Dr J can do nothing.

After the NSW AIDS legislation

Dr J can notify the Director of Health that he has reason to believe McW may be antibody positive. The Director may, if he thinks fit, order McW to have himself tested. If the result is positive McW now has a legal obligation to inform Mrs McW of this fact. If McW does not do this then his legal position becomes the same as that of Mr McG in Case 3.

Case 5

Jim and Ted meet in a sauna and go off to spend the night together. A few days later Jim is talking to Bill. He mentions that he has met Ted. 'I hope that's all there was to it,' says Bill. 'You know Ted is utterly irresponsible. He had the antibody test and found he was positive, but all that has happened is that he's become more reckless than ever.' Jim is shocked, then enraged. Ted had told him quite explicitly he was 'clear' and there was no need to worry. Jim goes to the police.

Before the NSW AIDS legislation

There is nothing the police would do for Jim since Ted has not done anything that they would recognise as being against the law.

After the NSW AIDS legislation

Since Jim's complaint is that Ted has done something which is against the law, the police may conduct an investigation. They may set about ascertaining whether Ted is in fact antibody positive. If he is and if Jim continues to claim that he was not appraised of the risks the matter could go to court.

SUMMING UP

The NSW AIDS legislation does make a difference. Individuals who are antibody positive and who engage in sexual intercourse without informing their partners of the risks involved will be liable to prosecution, even where there is no infection of the other party or, alternatively, it cannot be established that infection resulted from intercourse with that particular person. This means that an individual who, without consent, has been exposed to the risk of HIV infection through sexual intercourse now has some form of legal redress. It also means that a medical practitioner, who has access to information to which a party at risk does not, may then take steps which will result in a police inquiry. This inquiry may result in the party at risk being informed of the risk to which he or she is being subjected and could eventually lead to the courtroom.

HOW EFFECTIVE CAN WE EXPECT THE NSW AIDS LEGISLATION TO BE IN CURTAILING THE SPREAD OF AIDS?

From all that has now been said about the nature and practice of the criminal law it seems unlikely that there will be large numbers of convictions. It is doubtful that either the probability of being prosecuted or the severity of the penalty is sufficiently high to constitute a serious deterrent to would-be offenders. But then, as I argued in Chapter 5, it is implausible to view deterrence as the primary purpose of the criminal law. If, on the other hand, we accept that the purpose of the criminal law is to set limits to socially tolerable behaviour, it seems quite appropriate to enact legislation regulating sexual activity of the kind contained in the Public Health (Proclaimed Diseases) Amendment Act 1985.

DO WE NEED MORE RADICAL MEASURES?

There will, of course, be those who say that the NSW criminal law (even post-1985 AIDS legislation) is too weak an instrument for bringing to a halt the transmission of the HIV virus via sexually irresponsible behaviour, and that there should be tougher legislation. Once one begins to consider what this tougher legislation should be, one is immediately beset by all kinds of difficulties. To prohibit an antibody positive individual from having sexual relations with an antibody negative one, where the latter is appraised of the facts and nevertheless consents, seems to be unjustifiably paternalistic. (This subject will be discussed in the following chapter.) Any attempt to isolate or confine all sexually active antibody positive individuals so that they have no opportunity to interact sexually with antibody negative ones is not justified, since we cannot justify interfering with the morally responsible who constitute no threat to others.

IS THE PENALTY SUFFICIENTLY HIGH?

Some may object that the penalty proscribed for those convicted of sexually reckless behaviour under the NSW AIDS legislation is too light and should be harsher. But then we live in a country where the penalties for murder, rape and assault are comparatively light. In view of this it would be unfair to inflict more draconian punishments on those who break the law regulating the sexual behaviour of those infected with HIV. It is almost certain that a rape victim will suffer severe psychological distress as the result of his or her experience, and frequently there will also be serious physical harm. On the other hand, even with unprotected anal intercourse — the most risky of sexual practices — the probability that the HIV virus will be transmitted during any one act of intercourse is well below 50 per cent, and with vaginal intercourse the risk is much, much lower.

It is my view that the Public Health (Proclaimed Diseases) Amendment Act 1985 provides an appropriate means for dealing with those sane, adult HIV infected individuals who behave in a sexually irresponsible manner, thereby placing others at risk of infection. The facts that some will be discouraged from being tested because of this legislation and that the law will at times be difficult to enforce are real costs. But the benefits are substantial and, in my view, outweigh these costs. The legislation provides a measure of legal redress for persons who have been exposed to the risk of HIV infection because others have chosen to behave in a sexually irresponsible way. It also provides medical practitioners with a mechanism whereby they may take action when they have reason to believe that a patient is being exposed to risk of infection without consent.

THE OTHER STATES

The only states in Australia that have enacted legislation criminalising sexual activities likely to lead to the transmission of the HIV virus are NSW and Queensland. The law in the other states and territories remains as it was before the AIDS crisis. If Mr and Mrs McX (of Case 1) are residents of Victoria, South Australia, Western Australia, Tasmania or the Northern Territory, then Mrs McX's legal position will be essentially the same as it would have been in NSW prior to the introduction of the NSW Public Health (Proclaimed Diseases) Amendment Act of 1985.

Let us now suppose the McXs are residents of Queensland. Here the relevant piece of legislation is the Queensland Health Act Amendment Act (No.2) 1984, S54 (12).

> Any person who knowingly infects any other person with any venereal disease shall be liable to a penalty not exceeding $10 000, or to imprisonment for any period not exceeding two years, or both, unless at the time the infection was transmitted to the person so infected, the person so infected was the spouse of the first-mentioned person, or was in a connubial relation with the first mentioned person, knew that the first-mentioned person was at the time infected with the venereal disease in question and voluntarily ran the risk of being so infected.

If Mrs McX becomes antibody positive and makes a complaint to the police, the above legislation will provide them with grounds for conducting an investigation, and the matter could well go to court. If it does go to court then the verdict will depend upon

AIDS AND THE CRIMINAL LAW

whether (or not) it can be established that Mr McX knew he was infected with HIV, whether or not he informed Mrs McX of the fact that he was HIV infected (and she agreed to accept the risk), and whether or not it can be established that Mrs McX became HIV infected as a consequence of her sexual relations with McX. McX can only be found guilty if it can be established beyond reasonable doubt that it was he who transmitted the virus to Mrs McX, that he knew that he was infected, and that he did not warn Mrs McX of the risk she placed herself under in having sexual relations with him. As has been remarked earlier in this chapter, there may be significant problems in establishing whether a person has indeed informed his or her sexual partner of HIV infection. Similarly, establishing that Mrs McX became infected with HIV as a result of her sexual relations with McX may well be difficult — suppose, for example, that Mrs McX has had sex with other HIV infected persons during the relevant period of time.

The law in NSW differs from that in Queensland in that in NSW it is not necessary to establish that Mrs McX became infected with HIV as a consequence of her sexual relations with Mr McX in order to obtain a conviction. To obtain a conviction under the NSW Public Health (Proclaimed Diseases) Amendment Act of 1985, all that needs to be proved is that McX knew he was HIV infected, and had sex with Mrs McX without appraising her of the risk she thereby placed herself under.

A second and equally important difference between the NSW and Queensland laws with respect to the sexual transmission of HIV concerns the role of consent. John and Sally have an ongoing sexual relationship, though they are neither married nor living together. John discovers that he is antibody positive. He tells Sally. Having thought the matter over Sally decides that she is prepared to accept the risk that goes with continuing her sexual relationship with John. Some months later Sally has the antibody test and finds that she is now antibody positive.

For the sake of argument, let us suppose that Sally goes to the police and tells them that John has infected her with HIV. The police will interview Sally. In NSW, they will ask her whether John informed her of the fact that he was antibody positive, and whether she consented to undertake the risk of continued sexual relations with him. If Sally tells the truth and admits that John did inform her about the risks and that she agreed to take them, the matter will not go to court since, according to the NSW Public Health (Proclaimed Diseases) Amendment Act of 1985, if Sally has been informed of the risks and has agreed to take them then no offence has been committed.

On the other hand, if Sally and John live in Queensland the matter may still go to court. According to the Queensland Health Act Amendment Act (No. 2) of 1984 the question of Sally's consent becomes important *only* if she and John are married or living in a de facto relationship. Since Sally and John are not, the fact that John informed Sally of the risk and Sally consented to take that risk is irrelevant as far as the law in Queensland is concerned.

ADDITIONAL READING

Howie, R.N. and Webb, P.J. 'The Legal Response to AIDS' *The Australian Journal of Forensic Science* Vol. 18, No. 1, 1985
'Hyam V.D.P.P. (Lord Hailsham)' *All England Law Reports* London:1974, Vol. 2, 41 ff
Kirby, M.D. 'AIDS Legislation — Turning Up The Heat?' *The Australian Law Journal* Vol. 60, 1986
New South Wales Public Health (Proclaimed Diseases) Amendment Act, No. 183, 1985
Salmann, P. and Willis, J. *Criminal Justice in Australia* Melbourne: Oxford University Press, 1984

QUESTIONS

1 Why do you think the law requires that an individual be proved guilty *beyond reasonable doubt*? Does this make the standard of proof too high? If the choice is between letting some of the guilty go free and sentencing some of the innocent, which would you choose? Would you make the same choice in the case of all crimes? Compare murder, rape, fraud. What about tax evasion?
2 Do you think our legal penalties, in general, are too light, too heavy, or just about right? Do you think that relative to each other they are correct? Are there any anomalies? Take a case, say that of a rape or a murder, and compare the penalities here and those prescribed in the NSW AIDS legislation for the sexually reckless. Now consider the kinds

of penalities to which drunken drivers are subject. Does the situation seem equitable?

3 'Everyone knows that it's possible to catch AIDS if you are promiscuous. So if you sleep around then it's your own fault if you get AIDS. It's not necessary to have a law like the one NSW has.' Discuss.

7 Paternalism

BEN: Why are you late this morning?

JERRY: Oh, we got pulled over by the cops — Dad wasn't wearing his seatbelt.

ANNE: Did he get fined?

JERRY: Yes. And he was really mad about it. He went on for the rest of the trip about it being his life and therefore he should be able to do what he likes with it.

BEN: He has got a point there. After all, the police don't go around putting out people's cigarettes and we all know that smoking causes lung cancer.

ANNE: Well, maybe they should! Not literally, of course, but what I mean is maybe nobody should be allowed to sell cigarettes.

BEN: You've got to be joking! I suppose you'd also want to ban alcohol and stop people sky-diving or mountaineering or driving racing cars.

ANNE: Well, it would be better for them if they didn't. They're all high-risk activities and chances are you'll end up killing or seriously injuring yourself.

BEN: And so what? It's your life, you're entitled to do with it as you want. Why should someone else be able to decide for you what risks you are allowed to take? If I choose to go sky-diving and have an accident then I'm the one who pays the costs. It's no one else's business what I do.

JERRY: But do you pay the costs? If you get killed, maybe. But suppose you're seriously injured. Then if you don't have private health insurance it's all of us, or at least our parents, who pay the costs in their taxes. It's the same if you smoke and get lung cancer. The community ends up paying the costs.

BEN: Well then, why not ban all motor vehicles from the roads? That way there would be no car accidents and no car accident victims!

ANNE: You don't have to go that far, Ben. After all, there are huge benefits that go with having motor vehicles. We can all get to where we want to go quickly, get fresh food fast and all that.

BEN: Yes, I can see there is a difference. So let's go back to smoking, where there don't seem to be any equivalent large scale benefits. In our society there are costs the community ends up paying if I smoke and get lung cancer. But suppose there was no Medicare and we all had to pay our own medical bills. What would you say then?

JERRY: In that case I agree you should be free to smoke, go driving without a seatbelt or whatever.

ANNE: I don't think it makes the slightest difference. If it's clear that someone is going to be injured if he embarks upon some silly activity then the right thing is for society to be able to stop him doing it.

BEN: So you would have stopped Marco Polo going to China, or Captain Cook coming to Australia? And you'd close down the space exploration project.

ANNE: No, I wouldn't. Marco Polo and Captain Cook were on expeditions to discover more about the world. And it's the same now with space exploration.

BEN: Okay, I get the point. But you would have stopped Edmund Hillary from climbing Everest. After all, the top of any big mountain is much like the top of any other and it's not as though they are able to use the top of Everest for anything.

ANNE: When you describe it like that I suppose I'd have to say I don't think it should be allowed. But somehow...

BEN: Somehow you think climbing Everest is different from going sky-diving?

ANNE: Yes. Climbing Everest was an achievment because it had never been done before, but going sky-diving is just silly.

JERRY: But Anne, that just shows what your values are. Other people may have different ones.

In Chapter 4 I argued that in some circumstances discrimination against individuals, or groups of individuals, may be justified when the consequences of not discriminating are demonstrably worse than the consequences of discriminating.

Let's look now and see whether governmental interference with the liberty of an individual can ever be given a paternalistic justification. Is a government justified in interfering with the liberty of an individual to protect that individual from *himself or herself*? This is clearly a very different question from the one raised in Chapter 4 when we were concerned with consequences in general, that is, the consequences for *all* those affected by a particular policy or action. Supppose Fred has tuberculosis. One may argue that Fred should be removed from society at large until he is no longer infectious on the ground that to allow him to continue to wander freely about infecting others will result in consequences far worse than the admittedly unpleasant consequences he will suffer as a result of his quarantine. But one may also argue that Fred should be quarantined and treated — even if this is against his will — because to be cured of tuberculosis is in Fred's own objectively best interests. This argument, unlike the former, is a paternalistic justification for forcibly quarantining Fred.

Liberal philosophers usually start out with a presumption in favour of liberty. J.S. Mill, for example, argues that the only justification for interfering with the liberty of an individual is the prevention of harm to others. Paternalistic intervention — that is, intervention to protect the individual from himself — is not justified.

> .. the sole end for which mankind are warranted, individually or collectively, in interfering with the liberty of action of any of their number, is self-protection. That the only purpose for which power can be rightfully exercised over any member of a civilized community, against his will,

is to prevent harm to others. His own good, either physical or moral, is not a sufficient warrant. He cannot rightfully be compelled to do or forebear because it will be better for him to do so, because it will make him happier, because, in the opinion of others, to do so would be wise, or even right. (Mill, 1968: 72-3)

But having made this generalisation, Mill almost immediately steps back to make exceptions of various cases. Children are excepted, and so are idiots. One is even justified in interfering with a sane, adult individual where that individual is unaware that his actions are placing him at risk. Mill argues, for example, that one is justified in forcibly restraining an individual from crossing a dangerous bridge long enough to inform him of its (dangerous) condition.

Cases like these are cases of weak paternalism. Mill's individual about to cross the bridge is unaware of the risk he is about to take, and this justifies interfering with his progress in order to warn him of the risk. Similarly, the child who chooses to ride his skateboard on a busy highway may be regarded as not in a position to make a realistic assessment of the risks to which he will be subjected, simply because he is a child, and so too with the mentally retarded and the insane. With the man about to cross the bridge we can argue that if he were aware of its condition, he himself would freely choose not to cross. With the child we can argue that if he were older — that is, if he were possessed of a greater degree of mental maturity — he himself would recognise the danger in riding his skateboard on the highway, and would choose not to do it. With the mentally retarded person we can argue that he would not take various risks if he had normal intelligence, for then he would recognise the magnitude of those risks. And similarly with the person suffering from a mental illness.

But the issue which concerns us here is whether *strong* paternalism is ever justified. Is the state justified in coercing a mature, sane, intelligent individual to take a course of action that is (objectively) in his or her own best interests?

Before looking at this question there are one or two points which should be clarified. A policy or law is frequently given a *number* of different justifications. For example, the legislation which requires individuals to wear seatbelts is justified *both* in terms of the protection the seatbelt affords the seatbelted individual and the fact that since we have state-subsidised medical care, carelessness in this matter imposes an unfair burden on other taxpaying members of the community. Laws which prohibit cigarette advertising on television again are justified in many different ways. On the one hand they are justified on the paternalistic ground that individuals who are not exposed to such advertising have a better chance of staying non-smokers; *ergo* they have a better chance of living longer. On the other hand they are justified on the ground that, since the community pays for much of an individual's medical care, smokers hospitalised with smoking-related illnesses place an unfair burden on non-smokers. Multiple justifications for policies or laws is a common state of affairs and so it will nearly always be more accurate to describe a policy as having a paternalistic aspect, or a paternalistic justification.

John Stuart Mill is strongly anti-paternalistic. He argues that overall society would be better served if individuals were assured of a sphere of liberty into which the state would not intrude. Mill distinguishes conduct (or behaviour) that is self-regarding from that which is not, and argues that, in the case of the former, interference by the state cannot be justified. But what does Mill mean by self-regarding conduct, and how does self-regarding conduct differ from other-regarding conduct? Some have interpreted Mill's distinction as being one which divides actions which only affect oneself from actions which affect others. If we interpret Mill in this way very few actions will be truly self-regarding. Let's look at an example. Whether I choose to catch the 7.30 am or the 8 am train will have effects upon others, in so far as passengers who get on after me will have their chances of getting a seat augmented or diminished according to the course of action I adopt. So even the most trivial actions of an individual do have some trivial effects upon others. And for less trivial actions the effects may be more serious. Suppose I become an alcoholic. In this case the psychological and even physical welfare of my family may be adversely effected, and so the action of drinking a lot of alcohol is not self-regarding, because it does have effects upon others.

If self-regarding actions are actions which only affect oneself then Mill's individual cannot be guaranteed any significant sphere of liberty — a result which Mill certainly did *not* want. So let's look at another possible interpretation. Some have interpreted Mill as making a distinction between actions which affect the *interests* of others and actions which do not. This distinction differs from the distinction which divides actions into those which merely affect others and those which do not. Take the case of my choosing to catch the 8 am train. Because I catch this train rather than the 7.30 train Fred Bloggs who lives further down the line, and who also catches the 8 am train, does not get a seat. Fred has to stand up for the whole trip into the city. He has certainly been affected by my action, but it is not the case that any of his interests have been affected. Individuals can be said to have interests in such things as good health, adequate nutrition and sufficient education, but it is implausible to claim that they have an interest in anything so trivial as a seat on the morning train. So this latter interpretation allows us to dismiss the case of which train I catch since no fundamental interest of an individual is affected when his chance of getting a seat for his journey into the city is diminished. However, it is not similarly easy to dispose of the case of alcoholism. For here it *is* plausible to argue that the interests of, say, the alcoholic's children have indeed been adversely affected. A child's interests encompass such things as sufficient food, adequate housing, a stable environment, sufficient intellectual stimulation, and even a happy home. The unlucky child with an alcohol dependent parent may have any or all of these interests compromised.

Arguments such as these give rise to doubts as to whether there is any significant class of non-trivial actions which are truly self-regarding. But then maybe non-interference with some kinds of actions of individuals — those Mill referred to as self-regarding — can still be defended on the general ground that the costs associated with interference here outweigh the benefits.

A more direct attack on anti-paternalism is provided by those who argue that paternalistic interference may be justified because freedom is merely an *instrumental* good. An instrumental good is something that counts as good simply because it provides a means for obtaining some other valuable end or, in other words, a 'real' good. According to this argument, the non-instrumental or 'real' goods (ie food, clothing, companionship, sex, etc.) are what we should be seeking to augment. In so far as freedom facilitates the acquisition of such goods, it is itself a good. But only to this extent. If an individual is behaving in a way that is not in his or her own objectively best interests then paternalistic interference may be justified.

A variation on this argument recognises liberty as one of the 'real' goods. However, since an individual's liberty at a particular time may be augmented or diminished by actions he or she has taken at some earlier time, paternalistic interference at that earlier time may be justified on the ground that it will increase the individual's liberty at a later time.

Another related argument seeks to undermine the distinction between strong and weak paternalism. According to this view all paternalism is really weak paternalism. And since weak paternalism is justified, then paternalism is justified. This argument may be mounted in one of a number of forms. It may be argued that *in the future* the individual who is the object of paternalistic interference will come to consent to what he or she was previously coerced into doing. Or it may be argued that since the coerced action is the rational action, the individual, if he or she had been truly rational at the time, would have consented to it. His or her irrationality at the moment of decision justifies paternalistic intervention to enforce the rational option.

These kinds of arguments are open to two rejoinders. First, in presuming that the coerced individual will/would/should come to see (and accept) the correctness of the action forced upon him or her, we are accepting that there is some generally preferred ordering or set of tastes. But then there is very little evidence that this is so. Some individuals whose sanity is otherwise well demonstrated choose to spend a lifetime engaging in high risk activities — eg driving racing cars, climbing mountains, or parachuting from low altitudes. If we accept these choices as defensible, then it is difficult to rule out other risky activities like driving without a seat belt, smoking, or drinking to excess. That a preference is non-standard does not in itself establish that it is not a genuine preference.

Now for the second rejoinder. Even if it is the case that an individual will (or would) come to share the values that his or her coercer now has, this of itself does not establish that the values of the coercer are 'better' values. What grounds are there for assuming that the risk-averse individual is the highest form of human life? Few! If we take an Aristotelian or Sartrean view, and accept that we make our characters in making our choices, the individual who acts recklessly is in effect choosing to be one *kind* of individual rather than another. This choice may result in his or her becoming either a paraplegic or an adventurer of heroic proportions. But surely it is up to the individual to decide how he or she should live his or her life.

J.S. Mill, in making his case against paternalism, put forward a number of arguments. The first is a pragmatic argument that others are unlikely to choose for another individual as well as he or she would choose for himself or herself, because they will lack information about that individual's precise circumstances, and because they do not have to live with the choice made (whereas the other person does!). A second argument is that an individual restrained from choosing for himself or herself, and from living with the consequences of his or her own choices, will fail to develop. The act of choosing, and living with consequences of one's choice, is a vital ingredient in an individual's development.

Behind both these arguments is Mill's conviction — a conviction shared by most modern liberals — that the individual is entitled to some degree of protection from interference from others. People should not be viewed as a mere means to a more cosmic end, and affording the individual some degree of protection from the interference of others will result in a better society than will the alternative.

PATERNALISM, AIDS AND SEX

HIV is transmitted through sex and blood. Sexual intercourse may lead to the transmission of the HIV virus. Sharing infected syringes may have the same result. So would the state be justified, on paternalistic grounds, in enacting laws prohibiting uninfected individuals from having sex or sharing needles with infected ones?

Let us take a look at the Queensland legislation that is relevant to controlling the sexual transmission of the HIV virus.

> S 54 (12) *Infecting another with venereal disease.* Any person who knowingly infects any other person with any venereal disease shall be liable to a penalty not exceeding $10 000, or to imprisonment for any period not exceeding two years, or both, unless at the time the infection was transmitted to the person so infected, the person so infected was the spouse of the first-mentioned person, or was in a connubial relation with the first-mentioned person, knew that the first-mentioned person was at the time infected with the venereal disease in question and voluntarily ran the risk of being so infected. (Queensland Health Act Amendment Act (No. 2) 1984)

The major difference between this prohibition and its NSW equivalent is that the Queensland law constitutes a paternalistic interference with the sexual freedom of many sane, adult individuals. In NSW an HIV infected person — call him Fred — may have sexual intercourse with an uninfected person — call her Mary — provided Fred first tells Mary of the risk involved, and Mary agrees to take the risk. If Mary later becomes infected with HIV then Fred is not legally culpable. But in Queensland, if Fred and Mary are neither married nor living together, and Mary becomes infected as a consequence of having sex with Fred, then Fred can be fined $10 000, imprisoned for two years, or both. The fact that Mary knew about Fred's infection and decided to have sex with him anyway cannot be used as a defence by Fred. Of course it would have to be proved in a court of law that Mary became infected with HIV as a causal consequence of having sex with Fred. And for all the reasons set out in the last chapter this will frequently be something that is impossible to prove.

But regardless of whether there will be many convictions for transmitting HIV under this law, section 54(12) of the Queensland Health Act Amendment Act (No.2) 1984 is paternalistic. Admittedly Fred is the principal object of this law for it is he who will be subject to prosecution if Mary becomes infected. And certainly the law is not paternalistic with respect to Fred — Fred is prohibited from doing something which is potentially harmful to others. But the law is indirectly paternalistic, for, to put it crudely, it is a law which restricts Mary's access to sex. A law which prohibits the manufacture and sale of heroin is paternalistic with respect to potential customers because it restricts their access to heroin. This Queensland law is likewise paternalistic in that it limits the liberty of mature and sane individuals like Mary who are aware that there is a risk attached to having sex with someone like Fred but may still choose to take that risk.

Some have argued that paternalistic intervention is justified in those cases where there is a large differential between the magnitude of the restriction imposed and the magnitude of the benefit gained. An example of a restriction that fits this description is our seatbelt legislation. It has been argued that this piece of paternalistic legislation is justified on the ground that it is very non-restrictive to wear a seat belt, and one may be saved by this from becoming a paraplegic. The restriction is tiny, the potential benefits immense.

Can this kind of argument be used to justify the Queensland legislation we have been discussing? The answer to this question is no. Even if the line of argument were defensible in the case of seatbelts, it would not be applicable in the case of the sexual transmission of HIV. Sex is non-contentiously one of the central 'goods' in life, and sexual satisfaction is certainly more central to life than seatbelt-free drives through the countryside. Some individuals are more interested in sex than are others, and for those individuals for whom sex is not very important it would be silly to take the risk of becoming infected with HIV when the only benefit to be gained is another sexual experience. But there are also people for whom sex is very important, in fact so important that they are prepared to undertake significant risks in order to have it. As with many other things, the one best placed to decide for an individual what risks he or she is prepared to accept in order to obtain a valued end is that very individual. The individual is most likely to have most information about his or her own priorities, and therefore he or she is best placed to decide what level of risk is acceptable to him or her.

A similar state of affairs exists when religious commitment and health come into conflict. In this case the state is not permitted to intervene to ensure that a sane, adult person does what is best for his or her health. The state does not, for example, coerce a sane adult Jehovah's Witness to have a blood transfusion even though this may be medically imperative. The decision whether or not to have a blood transfusion belongs to the individual. Since sexual attitudes are at least as central to the individual as are his or her religious beliefs, the state therefore has no business coercing the individual to curtail his or her sexual activities in order to preserve his or her own good health. Similarly, moves to close gay bath houses and gay social institutions cannot be justified on paternalistic grounds.

People like Mary should be allowed to direct their own lives and decide what risks they are prepared to undertake in the pursuit of sexual satisfaction. Legislation of the kind that exists in NSW is to be preferred to its Queensland equivalent because, while the former prohibits reckless sexual behaviour that may spread HIV, it allows individuals, regardless of their domestic arangements, to decide for themselves whether they are prepared to undertake the risks involved in engaging in sexual intercourse with an HIV infected person.

PATERNALISM, AIDS AND DRUGS

Paternalistic interference in the life of a sane adult is not justified, but there are circumstances where it may be. One method of legitimising paternalistic intervention — and a method used by Mill — is to show that the agent in question lacks that rationality required for making a proper decision. Such failure of rationality may occur for any of a number of reasons — extreme youth, insanity, or, as is here relevant, a physical addiction.

The intravenous drug addict will typically behave in ways that appear grossly reckless to the non-addict. He or she will risk imprisonment and a criminal record in order to procure small sums of money through burglary. Women may go into prostitution — and take on its attendant risks — to the same end. But the intravenous drug user is not irrational in the sense that he or she is unable to see the consequences of his or her actions. He or she can see the consequences of his or her alternative possible actions quite clearly. It's just that from the addict's point of view, virtually any risk becomes acceptable if it is one which must be taken to get more of his or her drug. Without that drug, an addict will suffer the tortures of withdrawal and so whatever else it is, behaviour aimed at the avoidance of such suffering is not irrational.

A drug addicted individual and a non-addicted one are typically in asymmetric positions. The non-addicted individual when offered a drug will typically be able to *either* accept or decline. The addicted individual, on the other hand, will (unless he or she has just had a fix) *only* be able to accept. And this will be the case despite the fact that the person may know that he or she is endangering his or her life and health, and may wish to continue to live.

Addicted intravenous drug users are proper objects of paternalistic intervention to the extent that they are unable to give appropriate weight to the risks of contracting HIV by using dirty needles. The addicted individual may be internally coerced to behave in a way that exposes him or her to risk of HIV infection. The addict's position is similar to that of someone coerced with a gun, though in the case of the addict the coercion is internal, and reducible to his or her physiological dependence.

Paternalistic intervention to prevent drug users from exposing themselves to the risk of HIV infection may, in certain circumstances, be justified. But then what exactly can be done? Criminalising the sharing of hypodermic syringes would be utterly pointless, for if the risk of contracting HIV is impotent with respect to curtailing the practice of sharing needles, then so too will be the threat of a criminal action. Intravenous drug users already face the threat of criminal action by virtue of the fact that they are users! In Chapter 9 I will return to this question, but now before leaving the topic of paternalism and drugs let us consider a more radical suggestion.

THE CASE FOR LEGALISING INTRAVENOUS DRUG USE

Despite the fact that intravenous drug use is against the law, such prohibitions are not terribly effective. There were, according to conservative estimates, 20 000 heavy narcotic users in Australia in 1983. The typical heavy user spent between $80 000 and $100 000 a year on drugs. The revenue for this was raised in the main (75 per cent) by theft. Six hundred million dollars of the $1800 million worth of property stolen in 1984–5 went to finance narcotics purchases.

And these are not the only costs borne by the community. There are medical expenses, productivity losses and the cost of law enforcement. The user too is faced with additional costs by virtue of the fact that the intravenous drug market is a black market. These costs include a component of the inflated black market price, ignorance with respect to the purity of the product, and the risk of infection with serum hepatitis or HIV which results from the practice of sharing needles.

The costs associated with the black market in intravenous drugs to both the community at large, and the drug user in particular, are such that we should consider some alternatives. So let's look at the case for legalising intravenous drug use.

I have argued that paternalism is unacceptable when its objects are sane, adult individuals. It follows from this that if a sane adult chooses to become an intravenous drug user, then the state is not entitled to intervene and prevent him or her from doing so on paternalistic grounds. Nor, it seems, is there a case for criminalising intravenous drug use on the basis of its causing harm to others. The fact that an individual is an intravenous drug user *in itself* constitutes no harm to others. Furthermore it seems that drug-related crime is *an effect* rather than a cause of the fact that intravenous drug users must obtain their drugs on the black market at inflated prices, and so we could expect that many of the problems mentioned above would disappear if heroin could be obtained at a low cost over the counter.

A frequently voiced objection to the proposal that intravenous drug use be legalised is that it would lead to an increase in the number of intravenous drug users. However this *of itself* does not establish that we should not reform the drug laws. The point which must always be kept in mind is that intravenous drug users are citizens of the state. Their preferences and individual welfare are as important as the preferences and welfare of any other citizen.

A second and more serious objection is that reform of this

kind would probably result in an increase in intravenous drug use by *minors*. Clearly there would need to be provisions to ensure that minors were not allowed unrestricted access to intravenous drugs. In the case of minors, paternalistic intervention to restrict access is justified on the ground that minors lack the maturity to make a decision which may permanently lock them into drug addiction. The drug laws could be liberalised without moving to a situation where heroin was stocked on supermarket shelves. A state of affairs where heroin was obtainable either at low cost on prescription or free of cost to registered users would represent a significant change from the status quo.

The black market in intravenous drugs imposes significant costs on both the drug users and the community at large. The fact that HIV is transmitted via infected needles has simply added to those already substantial costs to produce a situation where serious consideration should be given to the value of retaining laws criminalising intravenous drug use. Once intravenous drug use was legalised it would then be a straightforward matter to require those supplying the drugs to provide disposable syringes with every sale.

ADDITIONAL READING

Brown, V.A. et al *Our Daily Fix* Sydney: Australian National University Press, 1986.
Marks, R. 'A Freer Market for Heroin in N.S.W.', *AGSM Working Paper Series*, November, 1985
Mill, J.S. 'On Liberty' in *Utilitarianism, Liberty, Representative Government* London: Everyman, 1968.
Queensland Health Amendment Act (No. 2) 1984, No. 103, S54(12)

QUESTIONS

1 What is paternalism? What is the difference between strong paternalism and weak paternalism? Give examples.
2 Why do most of us believe strong paternalism is acceptable when its objects are
   (a) children
   (b) mentally retarded people
   (c) insane people

3 What arguments are there in favour of strong paternalism?
4 What arguments are there against strong paternalism?
5 Our seatbelt legislation can be given a paternalistic justification? What other justifications can be given for it? Is it really justified?
6 Do you think individuals should be free to:
   (a) drive without seat-belts
   (b) go sky-diving
   (c) use heroin
   (d) use marijuana
   (e) use alcohol
   (f) expose themselves to the risk of catching AIDS

   If so why? If not, why not? Are your answers all the same? If they are, can you formulate a general principle that covers all the cases? If they are not, can you give a general principle that accounts for why you have treated them differently?

8 Homosex and Heterosex

Although both men and women can be homosexual, the law has chosen to involve itself in the issue of male homosexuality only, and the focus of this interest has been upon a particular kind of homosexual activity — namely, those acts which involve the insertion of the penis of one male into the mouth or anus of another male.

Feminists may well feel affronted that female homosexual activity — that is, lesbianism — has traditionally not even been accorded the recognition accorded by prohibition. Does the absence of a penis make it a sexual non-event for legislators and judges?

Lesbians are homosexual in the broad sense of the term. However, since the criminal law has concerned itself only with male homosexual activities, much of the debate about homosexuality has focused upon homosexuality in that more narrow sense. For ease of discussion in what follows I too will focus upon homosexuality in this narrower sense.

Homosexual sex is still a crime in a number of states of the United States of America, and in our own states of Queensland, Tasmania and Western Australia. The relevant sections of the Tasmanian penal code are the following:

S 122 Any person who
(a) has carnal knowledge of any person against the order of nature;
(b) has carnal knowledge of an animal; or
(c) consents to a male person having carnal knowledge of him or her against the order of nature, is guilty of a crime

S 123 Any male person who whether in public or private commits any indecent assult upon, or other act of gross indecency with, another male person, or procures another male person to commit any act of gross indecency with himself or with another male person , is guilty of a crime.

The Queensland legislation is similar although in Queensland an individual can be arrested for an act of gross indecency without a warrant.

> SS 208 Any person who
> (1) Has carnal knowledge of any person against the order of nature; or
> (2) Has carnal knowledge of an animal; or
> (3) Permits a male person to have carnal knowledge of him or her against the order of nature; is guilty of a crime, and is liable to imprisonment with hard labour for fourteen years.
>
> SS 211 Any male person who, whether in public or private, commits any act of gross indecency with another male person, or procures another male person to commit any act of gross indecency with him, or attempts to procure the commission of any such act by any male person with himself or with another male person, whether in public or private, is guilty of a misdemeanour, and is liable to imprisonment with hard labour for three years.
> The offender may be arrested without warrant.

In Western Australia, while it is required that the arresting officer have a warrrant, whipping is still on the statute books for these crimes.

> S 181 Any person who
> (1) Has carnal knowledge of any person against the order of nature; or
> (2) Has carnal knowledge of an animal; or
> (3) Permits a male person to have carnal knowledge of him or her against the order of nature; is guilty of a crime and is liable to imprisonment with hard labour for fourteen years, with or without whipping.
>
> S 184 Any male person who, whether in public or private, commits an act of gross indecency with another male person, or procures another male person to commit an act of gross indecency with him, or attempts to procure the commission of any such act by any male person with himself or with another male person, whether in public or private, is guilty of a misdemeanour, and

is liable to imprisonment with hard labour for three years, with or without whipping.

Until well after the end of World War II homosexuality was a crime in many western countries. Great Britian decriminalised homosexuality (when the acts occurred in private between consenting adults) in 1967. South Australia enacted similar legislation in 1972, Victoria in 1980, and New South Wales as recently as 1984.

This important change in British law followed on from a recommendation in the famous Wolfenden Report. In 1954 the British government set up a committee under the chairmanship of John Wolfenden to look into the possibility of decriminalising homosexuality. That committee recommended that homosexual acts that occurred in private between consenting adults should no longer be criminal offences.

Taking the classic liberal position expounded by John Stuart Mill, they argued that the state is only justified in interfering with individuals in order to prevent harm to others. Since homosexual acts occurring in private between consenting adults posed no harm to others they were, in the view of the committee, the business of no one but the individuals involved, and therefore should not be considered criminal offences.

It seems clear that homosexual acts in private between consenting adults involve no harm to others. And Mill's principle — that the state is only justified in interfering with the individual in order to prevent harm to others — also seems very plausible. So how could anyone be opposed to the decriminalisation of the homosexual acts in question? Not surprisingly, many did oppose decriminalisation. Indeed some individuals still do.

OPPOSITION TO HOMOSEXUALITY

Why are people opposed to homosexuality? There are two kinds of answer to this question. The first is a psycho-social one. Homosexuals are a minority. Most people are heterosexual. As frequently happens in this situation the minority is viewed as inferior. Moreover, since the sexual drive is one of the strongest and most basic of human drives, those who have non-standard drives or drives with non-standard objects are not only looked upon as inferior but viewed with open hostility by the majority. And entrenched community values serve to reinforce these more primitive responses.

The second answer to this question, and the kind of answer which is of interest to us here, seeks to unearth whether or not those individuals opposed to homosexuality can produce good reasons or rational arguments in support of their views. It is to this latter kind of argument that we shall now turn.

Let's start with two very bad arguments.

If homosexuality is decriminalised more young boys will be homosexually molested. Therefore any homosexual act should be a crime.

The first criticism that can be made of this argument is that there is no evidence that the decriminalisation of homosexuality leads to an increase in the number of cases of homosexual molestation of young boys. But even supposing, for the sake of argument, that it did, this would not of itself constitute a justification sufficient for outlawing all homosexual acts. Only a minority of homosexual acts are cases which involve the molestation of young boys, and we already have laws which prohibit adults from having any kind of sexual relations with those below a certain age.

Second, if one accepts that outlawing an action may reduce its incidence then one would have to at least consider outlawing a good many other actions not presently illegal. It is a fact, for example, that many young girls are heterosexually molested . But would this justify a law outlawing heterosexual sex?

The general point worth making here is that many, indeed most, activities may generate bad consequences. Allowing large numbers of people to drive motor vehicles results in a certain number of road accidents. But the fact that allowing the ordinary citizen to drive a motor vehicle has this negative consequence does not demonstrate that we should ban him from the roads.

People will be better off if they are forced to be heterosexual. Therefore all homosexual acts should be crimes.

There are two major problems with this argument. First, it seems *just plain false* that a homosexual will be better off if he is forced to live a heterosexual lifestyle. Take Tom. He is an ambitious young barrister who wants to go to the top of his chosen profession. Tom realises that it will be much more difficult, indeed maybe impossible, for him to achieve his ambition if he does not disguise the fact that he is homosexual. So he takes on all the trappings of a heterosexual lifestyle. He marries Helen, who is much younger than he and lacks any previous sexual experience. Tom and Helen produce the requisite two children. But Tom is discontented because his sexual preference is not for women. From time to time he picks up other men and has sex with them. After all, he can't afford to have it get about that he is homosexual, and that is the risk he would run if he chose to 'come out'. These anonymous sexual encounters provide Tom with transitory erotic satisfaction, but at the same time he feels guilty with respect to Helen. But then he always feels guilty with respect to Helen because he has always used her to create a facade of respectability. Helen too is unhappy. She feels that something is wrong. Since the conception of their two children Tom has lost all sexual interest in her. She feels that Tom no longer loves her. As she looks back at her life she begins to wonder whether he ever did.

As this tale demonstrates, it is improbable that any long term good will come about as a result of pressuring people to pretend to have a sexual preference they do not really have. Such individuals are being forced to live lies. Tom suffers because of the fact that he must keep up a veneer of being heterosexual. Helen suffers because she believes that Tom does not love her. And doubtless their children suffer too — it would be strange if they didn't given the major deceit going on around them.

Now for the second problem. Even if we were to accept that in some objective sense people would be better off (for example, they would be less likely to get AIDS) if they were forced to be heterosexual, this does not establish that the state is justified in coercing them to be so since, as I have argued in the preceding chapter, paternalistic interference in the lives of sane, intelligent adults cannot be justified. A homosexual act in private between consenting adults does not effect the interests of anyone but those adults involved, and therefore the state has no ground for interference.

A more sophisticated argument frequently advanced by opponents of homosexuality goes as follows:

- Homosexuality is unnatural.
- Therefore homosexual acts are morally wrong.
- Therefore homosexual acts should be illegal.

But is it true to say that homosexuality is unnatural? What do we mean by unnatural? One reply to this question is that an action is unnatural if it is against the instincts of the individual performing the action. But presumably homosexual sex is not against, but rather in accord with, the instincts of the homosexual. After all, it is not unreasonable to assume that individuals are inclined to follow their instincts in sexual matters.

Why some people are homosexual and others are heterosexual no one really knows. It has been argued by some that homosexuality is the result of environment; others believe it is caused by exposure to certain chemicals in the mother's womb, while others again theorise that it is genetically determined. But while they differ with respect to the cause of homosexuality, the supporters of all of these three competing views are in agreement that homosexuals genuinely prefer homosexual sex. Certainly it would be unnatural for a heterosexual to have homosexual sex — it would be against his instincts. And it would also be unnatural for a homosexual to have heterosexual sex — it would be against his instincts. But it is perfectly natural — in the sense that it is in accord with the instincts of the individual involved — for the homosexual to have homosexual sex. Given this interpretation of unnatural, it is simply incorrect to say that homosexual sex is unnatural for homosexuals.

If an action is unnatural only when it is not in accord with the instincts of the agent who performs it, then homosexual sex is not unnatural for homosexuals. But can we find some other sense of unnatural that allows us to make some sense of the statement: homosexuality is unnatural. Some have argued that since our primary purpose as biological organisms is reproduction (if there were no reproduction the species would die out) homosexuality is unnatural because it cannot result in reproduction.

It is certainly true that homosexual sex does not lead to reproduction. However, while it is true that a species will die out if less than a critical number of its members reproduce, it is not necessary that all members of a species reproduce to keep the species going. Take bees. The vast majority of bees never reproduce — indeed, they are incapable of reproducing. The worker bee spends all its life labouring to secure the survival of the hive, but it is sterile and never reproduces. It is not unnatural that it does not reproduce. It cannot reproduce — that is the way it is.

It could be objected here that while it may be natural for the sterile worker bee not to reproduce, male homosexuality is a very different matter since most male homosexuals are fertile and therefore biologically capable of fathering children. It is just that they are not inclined toward those activities which will result in the production of children and so the probability that they will sire children is reduced.

But are the two cases really all that different? The bee will not reproduce because it is physically incapable. The homosexual is unlikely to reproduce because his preferred sexual behaviour will not result in the production of offspring. Suppose now that this behaviour has a genetic basis, a supposition entertained by E.O. Wilson in his book *Sociobiology: The New Synthesis*. It is then plausible to argue, as Wilson does, that, under certain conditions, homosexual behaviour could raise the probability of an individual's genes getting into the next generation.

Families, that is, genetically related individuals, share a lot of common genes. If my sister has a child some of my genes will get into the next generation even if I never have a child. Now in most circumstances I will raise the probability of getting more of my genes into the next generation if I have children of my own. But it's not hard to think of exceptions to this generalisation. Imagine there was a severe famine. If both my sister and I have numerous children, none of them will have enough to eat and they will all die. But if I do not have any children and give all the food I can manage to find to her children, some of them may survive. And this means that more of my genes may make it to the next generation than would have if I had had my own children.

Wilson uses this kind of example to support the suggestion that homosexuality may well have a biological point. In situations of scarcity, families containing homosexuals may succeed in raising more offspring than families containing no homosexuals because in the former case there will be more resources to concentrate on fewer offspring. And if Wilson is correct this will of course undermine the view that homosexuality is unnatural, in the sophisticated sense of unnatural we are here talking about.

Not everyone believes that homosexuality is genetically determined. As I mentioned earlier, there are at least three different schools of thought on the subject. Let's look briefly at the other two. Some argue that homosexuality is a consequence of a particular kind of upbringing. They argue that the homosexual would have grown up to be heterosexual but for his unfortunate, aberrant, environment. This explanation likens homsexuality to insecurity or the lack of confidence that results from an inadequate upbringing.

Others, for example Professor G. Dorner from the Institute for Hormonal Research in East Berlin, have argued that homosexuality is a consequence of the foetus having had the misfortune to be exposed to abnormal chemical levels while in the womb. Dorner argues that if a male foetus is exposed to abnormally low levels of testosterone in the mother's womb it will grow up to have homosexual inclinations. This likens homosexuality to something like the thalidomide syndrome. During the early sixties a drug called thalidomide was prescribed to pregnant women suffering from morning sickness. Unfortunately the drug caused many of the foetuses to develop in an abnormal manner and the women gave birth to children with short, stumpy limbs.

If either of these latter explanations of the occurrence of homosexuality turns out to be correct then maybe some sense can be made of the thesis that homosexuality is unnatural. But where can we go from there? I shall now argue that even if it could be shown that homosexuality is unnatural this in itself does not establish that homosexual behaviour is morally wrong.

Let us for the sake of argument assume that some sense can be made of the claim that homosexuality is unnatural. Can we infer anything from this about the morality of homosexual behaviour?

If someone develops acute appendicitis then the natural outcome is for the person to die. What would happen if the person were from a primitive tribe living in the wild? It is profoundly unnatural to rush the patient into hospital, anaesthetise and operate upon him or her. But does this make operating on people with appendicitis wrong? Are surgeons committing moral wrongs each time they perform this kind of operation? Similarly, it is natural for a premature baby to die — that's what would happen if we did not have sophisticated humidity cribs. Are hospital staff doing something that is morally wrong whenever thay place a premature baby inside a humidity crib?

In both these cases we believe it would be morally wrong *not* to intervene in order to save the person's life. In performing the appendectomy the surgeon is doing what is morally right. In placing the infant in the humidity crib the hospital staff also do what is morally right.

A paraplegic who moves around in a wheelchair rather than by foot is moving about in a manner unnatural for a human being. But is the paraplegic doing something morally wrong when he or she moves off in his or her wheelchair? Diabetics who inject themselves regularly with insulin are employing unnatural means to prolong their lives. But are they at the same time doing something that is morally wrong? Would it be morally better for the paraplegic to spend his or her days confined to bed, and for the diabetic to die in a coma? Again, we believe not.

Some kinds of animals, say langur monkeys, live in packs where only the dominant male mates with the females. Other males accept their submissive position or are driven out or killed. In some primitive human societies similar institutions prevail. Powerful, older males monopolise all the females, and young or unimportant males get none. These societies live far closer to nature than we do. But should we conclude from this that their arrangements are morally superior to ours? We do not, nor should we.

That something is natural does not establish that it is morally right. Nor does the fact that a practice is unnatural show it to be morally wrong. So even if we assume that homosexuality is unnatural this does not of itself establish that it is morally wrong. More argument would be required.

IS HOMOSEXUAL SEX MORALLY WRONG?

Let's look at an example. Bill and Joe are homosexuals. They like each other, and want to have sex with each other. There is no reason why they should not — no pledges of monogamy to others, no AIDS etc. Is it wrong for Bill and Joe to have sex? How would a utilitarian answer this question? What about a rights theorist? There are of course many more moral theories then these, but let's for a start look at just these two.

According to the utilitarian it is wrong to perform an action if not performing it would produce better consequences than performing it. But given the way that I have set up this case — namely so that there are no bad consequences — and given the assumption that some good consequences will flow from their having sex — for example, Bill and Joe will be happier — then according to the utilitarian they do nothing that is morally wrong when they have sex with each other.

The rights theorist argues that an individual has a *prima facie* right to express his sexuality in that manner to which he is most inclined. Given the way in which I have set up this case — Bill and Joe are both homosexual and would like to have sex with each other, and no one else's rights are interfered with — the rights theorist, like the utilitarian, will say that Bill and Joe do nothing that is morally wrong when they have sex with each other.

DOES THE FACT THAT SOMETHING IS MORALLY WRONG OF ITSELF ESTABLISH THAT IT SHOULD BE ILLEGAL?

In Chapter 5 I argued that the fact that something is morally wrong does not establish that it should be made a crime. Many crimes, for example murder, rape and assault, are also moral wrongs. But it is not their moral wrongness that makes them crimes. There are also cases where a practice is morally wrong but the law does not (and should not) intervene. Telling lies and breaking promises are wrong but they are not illegal. And it would be a mistake to make these practices illegal because enforcement of the law would require intrusiveness into the lives of individuals on an unjustifiable scale. That something is morally wrong does not in itself establish that it should be made illegal. More work is required.

What I shall now do is examine one very famous argument that attempts to do just this. This argument is the one advanced by Lord Patrick Devlin. In 1958 Lord Devlin took issue with both the Wolfenden Report and John Stuart Mill. Devlin argued that 'harm to others' is not the only justification for state interference with the liberty of individuals. In Devlin's view a society is also entitled to act to protect itself from harm.

Can we make sense of the idea of harm done to a society that does not reduce to harm done to its individual members? Devlin argued that a society is constituted not just by its individual members but by a community of ideas. This is certainly correct — there is more to a society than the sum of its individual members. A group of discrete families or tribes who inhabit a geographical region but have nothing to do with each other is not a society. A group of individuals only becomes a society when its members become associated in various important ways. More specifically, a group of individuals only becomes a society when those individuals reach some fundamental agreement about how the society is to be organised and how its members are to behave.

Fundamental agreement concerning what is and what is not acceptable behaviour from the members of a society covers such things as general consensus that rape, murder and theft are wrong, whereas caring for one's children or one's aged parents are moral duties. Agreement about these or similar matters constitutes what Devlin describes as the shared morality of the society.

Devlin accepts that the purpose of the law is to set the limits to socially tolerable conduct. He is interested in morality, or rather what he describes as the shared morality of the society, because under certain circumstances it provides a guide to what is socially tolerable conduct. What is particularly interesting about this argument is that it does not rely upon an assumption that the moral precepts in question, which will usually be those of a particular religion, are the correct moral principles. It has sometimes been argued that homosexuality ought to be a crime because it is against the law of God. (The Right to Life movement use this same argument against abortion.) The problem, however, is that deciding whether or not God exists is of its nature a difficult task. And even among those who accept that God does exist there is a great deal of disagreement about what are the laws of God. Devlin neatly sidesteps these difficult questions. All that his argument requires of his moral principles is that they be ones to which the members of the society are committed.

So let's now take an example, in fact an example which Devlin himself discusses. In both England and Australia the Christian notion of marriage, that of marriage being a permanent, monogamous union, constitutes part of our shared morality. This notion of marriage forms the basis of the kind of family life which exists in our society, and as such is an important determinant of the kind of society we have. Our laws, in forbidding polygamy and requiring divorce prior to remarriage, reinforce this particular notion of marriage. In Saudi Arabia the notion of marriage is rather different. Polygamy is an accepted institution, and this makes for a rather different kind of society.

Devlin is correct when he argues that changes in the law have the potential to alter the nature of the society in significant ways. Imagine for example that our bigamy laws were rescinded. Presumably a number of people would take advantage of the situation and acquire multiple spouses, and with the passage of time this would bring about important changes in family life and thus changes in the fundamental nature of the society.

But does the fact that change in the law may lead to social change, even fundamental social change, mean that our laws should never be altered? At this point Devlin's argument becomes rather more complex. Devlin's bottom line is that societies have a right to protect themselves. He also believes that anything that loosens the bonds of the shared morality of the society must be viewed as a potential threat to the existence of the society. But Devlin is not set upon ruling out all legal reform; his argument is more sophisticated than that.

Devlin makes a distinction between changes which are 'merely changes' and those which are potentially lethal to a society. Liberalisation of the law with respect to using marijuana or changes in the laws of inheritance to accommodate situations which may result from the 'test-tube baby' technology are (arguably) 'merely changes'. On the other hand, a change in the law that allowed tax evaders to go unpunished is (arguably) potentially lethal.

Devlin also differentiates between actions which the society at large views with 'intolerance, indignation and disgust' and actions of which the society may disapprove but with less vehemence. Adultery, in so far as it threatens the stability of the family, is according to Devlin potentially lethal to a society, but Devlin does not believe that there should be criminal sanctions against adultery since though the citizenry at large may view adultery as morally wrong they do not view it with 'intolerance, indignation and disgust'. Homosexual acts, on the other hand, are viewed with 'intolerance, indignation and disgust' and therefore, according to Devlin, should be illegal.

Devlin's position then is that the law may impose sanctions to enforce a piece of the shared morality of a society if the actions in question pose a threat to the existence of the society, and the society at large views the actions in question with 'intolerance, indignation and disgust'.

The first criticism which can be made of Devlin's argument is that even in Britain in the 1950s it would have been unrealistic to suppose that the decriminalisation of homosexuality could bring about the collapse of the society. Homosexuality is, and always has been, a minority preference. Adultery, on the other hand, has a direct impact on the stability of the family unit. If one takes seriously Devlin's claims that a society has a right to protect itself, and so preserve the kind of family life it has been built on, one must view adultery as a far greater threat to society than homosexuality. To dismiss the suggestion that adultery should be a crime on the ground that the majority of citizens do not view adultery with 'intolerance, indignation and disgust' leads one to suspect that Devlin's argument, in the final analysis, comes to nothing more than the claim that the majority (the heterosexuals), because they are a majority, have a right to tyrannise the minority (the homosexuals).

As we saw in Chapter 2 in our discussion of utilitarianism, allowing the preferences of a majority to determine the fate of the members of a minority group will give rise to all manner of undesirable states of affairs. The kind of argument used by Devlin against the decriminalisation of homosexuality could equally be used by an apartheid state to justify its racist policies. If the white majority think interracial marriage is morally wrong and view such alliances with 'intolerance, indignation and disgust' then, according to Devlin's argument, the state is justified in making interracial marriage a crime. Such implications should cause us to have grave doubts about Devlin's argument.

There have been many important social changes in the past 30 years. De facto spouses and illegitimate children are no longer ostracised by society. Whether or not to marry is properly considered to be a matter for each individual to decide for himself or herself. Similarly whether a woman chooses to work or stay at home is seen as being a matter of individual choice. Conservatives decry these changes, and some claim that society is falling apart, but it is hard to sustain the thesis that things are any worse than they were in times gone by. After all, women, who constitute 50 per cent of the population, do seem to be significantly better off. Things have certainly changed a lot since the 1950s and despite these changes there has been no real disintegration of the society.

Change for the sake of change is not a good thing, but neither is no change for the sake of no change. The conservative view that change has its costs is correct. But this does not show that there should never be change since failure to change may have greater costs. Each proposed reform must be looked at on its own merits and evalutated according to those merits. Should abortion be available upon demand? Should intravenous drug use be legalised? Should homosexuality be decriminalised? Should there be a market in human babies? All these issues should be debated and decided according to the merits of the particular case.

It is now the year 1988 and Britain has survived despite the fact that homosexuality was decriminalised over twenty years ago. Residents of NSW, Victoria and South Australia also live in states where homosexuality has been decriminalised and these states have not disintegrated as a result. Indeed it is difficult to see that there is any fundamental difference between the social fabric of these states and that of Queensland, Tasmania and Western Australia where homosexual acts are still crimes.

Homosexual acts in private between consenting adults do not

affect the interests of anyone but the individuals involved. They comprise no threat to the existence of the society. 'Pressuring' homosexuals to adopt heterosexual lifestyles can be expected to give rise to bad consequences for both the homosexual and his family. The case for according homosexuals the same rights as heterosexuals to express their sexuality is overwhelming.

ADDITIONAL READING

Dawkins, R. *The Selfish Gene*, Oxford: Oxford University Press, 1976
Devlin, P. *The Enforcement of Morals* London: Oxford University Press, 1965
Goldwyn, E. *The Fight to be Male* London: BBC (video), 1979
Mill, J.S. 'On Liberty' in *Utilitarianism, Liberty, Representative Government* New York: Everyman,1968
Wasserstrom, R. *Morality and The Law* Belmont California: Wadsworth, 1971
Wilson, E. O. *Sociobiology: The New Synthesis* Harvard: Harvard University Press, 1975

QUESTIONS

1 What is homosexuality?
2 What is heterosexuality?
3 Why do you think many people have a prejudice against homosexuality? List some of the arguments these people make? Do you think these arguments are valid?
4 Make a list, of at least 10 items, of acts which are natural but are morally wrong.
5 Make a list, of at least 10 items, of acts which are 'unnatural' but are morally right.
6 In the light of your answers to questions 4 and 5, what can we say about the statement, 'If something is natural that makes it morally right.'?
7 What was Devlin's argument against decriminalising homosexuality? What do you think of it?
8 Are there any advantages in pressuring homosexuals to pretend to be heterosexual? Are there any disadvantages
  (i) for the homosexual himself?
  (ii) for his family?
  (iii) for the community?

9 Prisons, Drugs and Kids

In Chapters 5 and 6 I argued that the criminal law is the most appropriate method for dealing with sane, adult, HIV infected individuals who behave in a sexually irresponsible manner. In this chapter I will look at some other cases where HIV infected individuals may pose a threat to others. These cases are all similar in that the individuals in question, like the sexually irresponsible person, cannot be relied upon to behave responsibly. However, these individuals differ from the sexually irresponsible person in that their lack of responsibility results from a mental incapacity or immaturity rather than being the result of choice. I will examine in turn the case of the mentally ill person infected with the HIV virus, that of the HIV infected drug user, and that of the HIV infected child. I will conclude the chapter with a discussion of the special problems raised by AIDS within prisons.

THE MENTALLY ILL PERSON

Individuals may be mentally ill independently of becoming infected with the HIV virus, or, on the other hand, they may become mentally ill as a result of their HIV infection. As I mentioned in Chapter 1, we now know that the HIV virus directly attacks the central nervous system. Some experts, including Dr Paul Volberding, head of AIDS services at San Francisco General Hospital, believe that those infected individuals fortunate enough to escape AIDS and ARC will all eventually succumb to the virus' direct attack upon the brain (Hancock and Carim, 1986: 28). Some of these individuals will suffer dementia, others will present with severe personality disorders or the symptoms of manic depression or schizophrenia.

What conditions must be met before a mentally ill individual can be detained in a mental institution on a non-voluntary basis? Let's look at an example.

The New South Wales Mental Health Act of 1983 allows for the involuntary detention of a mentally ill person within a hospital where a suitably constituted tribunal determines that detention of that person is necessary for the protection of others. Most importantly, before it is possible to detain a person on this ground it must be established that one of the following conditions has been satisfied.

(i) owing to the person's mental illness, the person has recently inflicted or attempted to inflict or has recently made a reasonably credible threat to inflict serious bodily harm upon another person;

(ii) owing to the person's mental illness, the person has recently performed or attempted to perform an act of violence, whether against a person or against property, which indicates that it is probable that the person will inflict serious bodily harm upon another person;

(iii) owing to the person's mental illness, the person has recently performed an act, engaged in a course of activity or constructed or set up a device or arrangement which will probably result in the infliction of serious bodily harm upon another person; or

(iv) owing to the person's mental illness, the person has recently engaged repeatedly in a course of behaviour of nuisance or harassment affecting one or more persons which would be reasonably likely to lead to violence and which is of a degree so far beyond the limits of normal social behaviour that a reasonable person would consider it intolerable. (NSW Mental Health Act, 1983, No. 178, 5. (1) (b))

What this means is that the mere possibility that a mentally ill person may cause harm to others is not sufficient to allow for his or her involuntary detention. The fact that most individuals suffering from that person's mental illness do satisfy one (or more) of (i) to (iv) is likewise not sufficient to allow that he or she be involuntarily detained. The individual *himself or herself* must satisfy one (or more) of (i) to (iv).

There are good reasons for this law being as it is. To begin with it is very difficult to predict precisely how an individual with a particular mental illness will behave in the absence of a lot of very particular information about the individual. In the second place it seems unjust to be able to forcibly detain and intern a mentally ill individual simply on the basis that he or she *may* constitute a threat to others where there is no real evidence of such a threat. Compare this situation with that of a sane individual. The criminal law allows for the detention of the sane individual only *after* he or she has committed a crime. The mere fact that he or she may do so, or even evidence that it is highly probable that he or she will cause serious harm to others, is insufficient ground for detaining the individual. Considerations of equity require there be some parity with respect to these two kinds of case.

One example of a psychosis which would render an agent likely to engage in actions that may lead to the infection of other individuals with HIV, and simultaneously render the agent not responsible for those actions, is manic depression. While in the manic phase individuals may be subject to overpowering sexual urges. They may also have delusions about their own powers and abilities, and become prone to gross recklessness. Manic depressives, typically, find it difficult to sustain personal relationships because during a manic phase they are prone to do things like spend all the family savings or give away the car. These days many manic depressives are successfully controlled with drugs, but some do not respond to this treatment, and others cannot be relied upon to take their medications.

Of course not all of these individuals constitute a threat to the health of others. In the first place most will not be infected with the HIV virus. But what of those who are HIV infected? Here again psychiatric opinion is that we can make no real generalisations. Some manic depressives will, during a manic phase, behave in a highly promiscuous manner. Others are either not subject to strong sexual urges or, alternatively, will repress them. So even for the class of HIV infected manic depressives in an uncontrolled manic phase we cannot say with certainty (or anything approaching it) that all members of this class constitute a theat to the health of others. What the law in NSW provides, however, is a legal mechanism whereby those who suffer from a mental illness, are HIV infected, and do constitute a threat to the health of others may be involuntarily detained.

The New South Wales Mental Health Act of 1983 also allows for the involuntary detention of a mentally ill person within a hospital where a suitably constituted tribunal determines that detention of that person is necessary *for his or her own protection*. However, before a person may be detained one of the following conditions must be satisified.

(i) owing to the person's mental illness; the person has recently attempted to kill himself or herself or to cause serious bodily harm to himself or herself;

(ii) there are reasonable grounds for believing that, owing to the person's mental illness, it is probable that the person will attempt to kill himself or herself or attempt to cause serious bodily harm to himself or herself;

(iii) there are reasonable grounds for believing that, owing to the person's mental illness, it is probable that the person will suffer serious bodily harm due to neglect of himself or herself or to neglect by others;

(iv) owing to the person's mental illness, the person has recently performed an act, engaged in a course of activity or constructed or set up a device or arrangement which will probably result in the infliction of serious bodily harm upon himself or herself; or

(v) the person is in the manic phase of a manic-depressive illness and there are reasonable grounds for believing that it is probable that the person will thereby suffer serious financial harm or harm to his or her reputation or standing in the community. (NSW Mental Health Act, 1983, No. 178, 5. (1) (b))

In Chapter 7 I argued that paternalistic interference may be justified in the case of mental incompetence. Thus the mentally ill person who is not infected with the HIV virus but who, if unrestrained, would be likely to become so is an appropriate object for paternalistic interference. The NSW Mental Health Act of 1983 already provides the legal mechanism to effect this policy — the individual may be detained under section 5. (1) (a) (iii).

The problems associated with the mental patient who is also HIV infected do not end with his or her institutionalisation. Within the psychiatric institution patients infected with HIV who are violent or sexually disinhibited may pose a threat to other patients or members of the hospital staff. An HIV infected patient who is attacked or has sexual attentions forced upon him or her may transmit the virus to his or her 'attacker'. In its guidelines for the management of AIDS and AIDS related disorders in psychiatric institutions the AIDS Task Force recommends routine antibody testing at the time of admission for all individuals belonging to high risk categories. It also suggests that it may be necessary to increase the supervision of HIV infected patients, and at times to segregate them.

INTRAVENOUS DRUG USERS

Intravenous drug users at present comprise the second largest category of AIDS victims. Using intravenous drugs does not in itself put one at risk of catching the HIV virus. Intravenous drug users are at high risk of catching the HIV virus because of the custom among them of sharing needles and syringes. An intravenous drug user who is not infected with the HIV virus but shares needles and syringes is placing himself or herself at risk of becoming infected. An intravenous drug user who is infected with the virus and shares needles and syringes is exposing others to risk of infection. The sexual partners of an HIV infected intravenous drug user may also be at high risk of becoming infected if the relevant precautions are not taken.

Prevention of the transmission of the HIV virus via infected needles can only be achieved if intravenous drug users stop sharing syringes. Unfortunately, there are two factors which encourage sharing needles. The first is the lack of availability of new disposable syringes. The second is the existence of a tradition among intravenous drug users that sharing syringes is part of the ritual surrounding such drug use. Educative materials stressing the dangers of HIV infection and promoting the use of clean syringes may have some beneficial effects, but such measures can be expected to achieve only limited success if users are unable to acquire supplies of sterile syringes.

Technically speaking, pharmacists who sell syringes to users are liable to prosecution. Since intravenous drug use is a crime in all Australian states and territories, a pharmacist who supplies a user with syringes may be charged with being an accessory to that crime, or of aiding and abetting that crime. I have already argued (in Chapter 7) that there is a strong case for decriminalising intravenous drug use. For the moment, however, let us ignore that more fundamental issue and concentrate on the question of whether pharmacists should supply users with new syringes.

Whatever one's attitude to drug use, one thing seems clear. It is worse for an individual to be both an addict and infected with the HIV virus than to be merely addicted. And the costs to society are greater too. If an individual is infected with HIV there is a high probability that he or she will in time succumb to AIDS or ARC and therefore require expensive medical treatments. Furthermore, each drug user who is HIV infected adds to the size of the pool of individuals who constitute a source of potential infection to others.

The case here is compelling. Pharmacists should be able to sell syringes to intravenous drug users, without fear of legal penalties. In some states this is already happening. In response to the AIDS crisis, programs are being set up in Western Australia, South Australia, NSW, Victoria and the ACT to allow drug users easier access to sterile syringes. These programs include the provision by pharmacists of low cost syringes, and 'exchange' programs where intravenous drug users can swap an old syringe for a packet of new ones.

The fact that intravenous drug users are now able to obtain new disposable syringes at a low cost over the counter has not, in NSW at least, induced many to avail themselves of this service. Some reports suggest that users consider the price ($2.40 for a pack of 5) to be too high. 'Exchange' programmes have been more successful, but it is estimated that a large number of drug users continue to share needles.

Despite educational programs and measures to allow drug users access to clean syringes, a significant number of them cannot be relied upon to behave responsibly and not share needles. And so, in this case, discriminatory treatment would seem justified.

What kinds of measures should we take? This will depend upon whether those who are behaving in an irresponsible manner can be considered responsible for their actions. In the case of the addicted individual, at least, it is plausible to argue that the judgement of such an individual is negatively affected. If this is so then measures similar to those already in place for dealing with the mentally ill would seem most appropriate. It should be possible to detain on a non-voluntary basis intravenous drug users who are infected with HIV and are either sexually irresponsible or likely to share needles. Similarly, this time on paternalistic grounds, it should also be possible to detain individuals who are not infected but whose own health is endangered as a consequence of their reckless behaviour.

But what of those cases (if there are any) where the judgement of the drug user is *not* impaired? Such an individual should be dealt with in the same way as the non-drug-using HIV infected individual who chooses to behave in a sexually irresponsible manner and so exposes his or her sexual partners to risk of infection. I argued in Chapters 5 and 6 that it is right that these irresponsible individuals be subject to legal sanctions, and so if HIV infected IV drug users, knowing they are infected, continue to share needles an equivalent case can be made for legal sanctions.

HIV INFECTED CHILDREN

Eve Van Grafhorst was an Australian preschooler who rose to national prominence as a consequence of her infection with HIV. Eve became infected as a result of receiving blood transfusions after her premature birth. Unfortunately for Eve that fact that she was antibody positive became public knowledge in her home town of Gosford when a local doctor 'leaked' this information to the town council.

Eve was excluded from her preschool, but was later readmitted at the Health Department's insistence. At this time most other parents chose to remove their children from the preschool. Within a few weeks, the decision regarding Eve was reversed when she bit another child, for now the Health Department claimed that Eve's behaviour made her a threat to other children. The Eve Van Grafhorst problem was finally 'solved' when her parents returned to New Zealand (her mother's native country) where Eve attends the local school without opposition from other parents.

In the United States there have been, to date, nearly 600 documented cases of children with AIDS, and the United States Public Health Service estimates there are over 2000 sick with HIV associated infections. By 1991 it is expected that this number will be in excess of 10 000.

THE NEW YORK CITY AIDS CASE

On September 7 1985 the mayor of New York City, Ed Koch, announced that a committee of experts had decided to allow a seven-year-old child infected with the HIV virus to attend a New York public school. Many parents responded by keeping their children at home and marching in the streets in protest. Subsequent to this, two community school boards brought actions against New York City, the Board of Education and the Health Department. Their aim was to have the infected child removed and to prohibit other infected children from attending public schools.

The lawyers and witnesses for New York City argued that the risks involved in allowing such a child to attend school were negligible. After all, transmission of the virus requires the exchange of body fluids. Normal social interaction with those infected with the virus is perfectly safe. Lawyers and witnesses for the city argued that children also faced risks when they caught the school bus or participated in athletic activities. Indeed there even existed a theoretical possibility that the roof of a classroom could fall in and kill a child. These risks certainly existed but they were so small that it would be foolish to eliminate athletic activities, make all children walk to school or take the roofs off classrooms.

The lawyers and witnesses for the schools boards, on the other hand, argued that there were possible (if not probable) interactions between children which could lead to transmission of the virus. An example of such an interraction is exchanging blood in 'blood-brother' rituals. They also argued that the expert witnesses for the city were only prepared to say it was *extremely unlikely* that children could be infected by others in classroom situations, but these witnesses were not prepared to say that it was *impossible* for one child to transmit the virus to another, and this was what parents were entitled to have guaranteed.

The HIV infected child, like any other child, will have much to gain from both the educational and social aspects of the school situation. On the other hand, each one of the other children with whom the infected child comes into contact will be at some (at this time still unquantified and certainly very small) risk of contracting the virus. [Obviously this problem is only significant with respect to younger children, who in the normal run of things will suffer minor cuts and abrasions, may bite each other, and do not always consistently follow the highest standards of hygiene.] But the problem is complicated by the fact that informing an HIV infected child that he may in certain circumstances be a threat to others could be expected to have serious psychological consequences for the child. Even if this were done it is unreasonable to expect that a young child would curtail his activities in an appropriate manner. After all, he or she is only a child!

As the lawyers for the State of New York argued, children, like all of us, are constantly at risk of injury from many sources. These risks may not be high but they do exist. We all risk injury and death, and impose risks of injury and death upon others whenever one of us drives a car down a street. Activities like riding horses or playing football also involve risks. Adults who engage in these activities voluntarily undertake these risks. Parents who allow their children to engage in these activities allow those children to be exposed to those risks. We do not usually brand such parents irresponsible. It is the general view within our society that if a sporting activity is properly supervised and reasonable care taken, the advantages — both physical and psychological — which accrue to those children participating in it outweigh the minor risks to which they are simultaneously subjected.

There are, of course, other activities that parents or schools will not allow children to engage in because they are considered to be too dangerous. Classes using swimming pools are usually not allowed unrestricted use of the high diving board. And children, generally, are not permitted to sky dive.

For parents of children mixing with an HIV infected child, however, the situation is one where whatever the magnitude of the risk to which their child is exposed there is, unlike swimming or football, no obvious countervailing gain. So why should parents let their children be exposed? The only advantage, it would seem, is to the infected child.

Let's now compare this risk to another. Every year a number of children drown in private swimming pools despite stringent safety requirements. One way to prevent these deaths would be to prohibit backyard pools. This is not done, though the existence of these pools constitutes an (admittedly very small) risk to children. So some risks to life, and more specifically in this case, risks to the lives of children are taken to be acceptable risks. The fact that a parent is unhappy about accepting the risk imposed on his child by others having private pools gives him no leverage.

There will be hardliners, like the attorneys and witnesses for the school boards, who maintain that no risk is acceptable, and that antibody positive children (and perhaps all people infected with the HIV virus) should be subject to strict discrimination. Then the question must be raised: why be so intolerant of this risk and simultaneously accept other risks of the same magnitude? Put another way, why discriminate against one particular kind of risk?

In the AIDS controversy in New York City the judge ruled that the child could not be excluded on the basis of existing health regulations. He went on to justify his decision by stating that the court was bound to evaluate the issue according to the evidence, and could not be influenced by irrational fears of catastrophe. With respect to this latter justification what the judge was doing was claiming that a *mere possibility* of harm resulting to others did not justify exluding the child. That some parents did not want to accept this risk was simply beside the point.

At the time of the New York City AIDS judgement there were no documented cases of infection with HIV resulting from accidents involving only skin-surface exposure to contaminated blood. In May 1987, however, the US Center for Disease Control issued a statement to the effect that there was now evidence that HIV could be transmitted as a result of skin-surface exposure to HIV infected blood. There were three cases: the first where blood seeped through the gauze covering the insertion site of an arterial catheter onto the chapped and ungloved hand of a nurse, the second where blood from an HIV infected patient splattered the face and mouth of a laboratory worker who was filling a vacuum flask with blood, and the third where a blood separating machine malfunctioned splashing the worker's ungloved hands and forearms with blood.

These cases are clearly relevant to class and schoolyard situations for they provide some empirical support to the fears of parents who believe that their children are at risk when they interact with an HIV infected child. Maybe thus it will be necessary to take precautions over and above the usual when a classroom contains a child infected with the HIV virus. But what precautions?

Let us now look again at the swimming pool analogy. The risk that a child will drown in a private pool can be lessened if parents are vigilant and pool owners fence their pools. And this is what (morally) responsible pool owners and parents will do to lessen the risk of any child drowning in a pool. Is there anything similar that the parents and teachers of HIV infected children may be able to do to lower even further the risk of one school child passing HIV on to another?

It is not possible for a teacher to take 'extra' precautions to prevent transmission of HIV in the classroom or schoolyard if the teacher does not know that a child is infected with the HIV virus. But if the teacher does know then the school may take appropriate action if any accidents occur which have the potential to lead to the transmission of the virus. The school may also supply extra supervision for certain activities like body contact sports. An obvious suggestion therefore is that the parents of an HIV infected child should inform the school about the child's HIV infection. Clearly there would need to be strict confidentiality requirements with respect to this information for otherwise the child could be victimised. If confidentiality could be guaranteed then the very greatest care could be exercised to ensure that other children were not exposed to the risk of infection while at the same time the child infected with the virus could reap the benefits — both intellectual and social — of a normal school environment.

AIDS AND PRISONS

As is the case outside, the primary modes of transmission of HIV within prisons are via sex and the sharing of infected needles. For obvious reasons, however, there are no accurate estimates of the amount of sexual activity that occurs between prisoners, nor of the amount of intravenous drug use that occurs there.

One suggestion for lowering the incidence of the sexual transmission of HIV within prisons would be to provide prisoners with access to condoms. There is no legal impediment to doing this in states where homosexuality has been decriminalised since there is nothing in the law prohibiting sex within prisons.

The main objection raised against this suggestion is that what evidence there is indicates that there is a high incidence of homosexual rape within prisons and therefore the supply of condoms could lead to an increase in its occurrence. It seems unlikely that the supply of condoms could be expected to increase the number of prison rapes for that would require the improbable scenario in which the rapist took time out to put on a condom!

In NSW, a decision to supply condoms to prisoners has still not been put into effect because of an industrial dispute concerning who is to distribute them. No other state has got as far as this. In those states where homosexuality has not been decriminalised the problem is very complex. Here it cannot be argued that prisoners are being unfairly disadvantaged with respect to the community as a whole when they are not provided with the means for having safer homosexual sex since it is illegal for anyone, prisoner or non-prisoner, to participate in such activities.

It can be argued, as I have done in Chapter 8, that the law which prohibits homosexual relations is an unjust law. The problem of the transmission of AIDS is sufficiently serious that one would hope it would lead states where homosexuality is still a crime to reform their laws. However the gravity of the situation is such that it warrants the supply of condoms to prisoners even in the absence of such law reform.

The problem of the transfer of HIV via infected needles within prisons is even more complex. As the law stands intravenous drug use is prohibited both inside and outside prisons. However, in response to the health problems generated by AIDS, it is now easy in some states at least for drug users outside prison to buy syringes over the counter, or exchange used syringes for new ones. Given that this is the case and that there is no special provision denying prisoners the right to obtain syringes, there should be no technical impediment to allowing prisoners access to clean syringes.

An important objection that has been voiced to this proposal is that prisoners could use these syringes as weapons. The case of the Sydney man who threatened a policeman that he would 'give him AIDS' provides substance to this fear. Supplying syringes to prisoners could well result in a situation of danger for both wardens and the less dominant members of the prison community.

So what else can be done? South Australia has recently decided to introduce compulsory antibody testing for all new prisoners and 70 per cent of those already imprisoned have voluntarily had the test. Under the new measures prisoners found to be antibody positive will be segregated from the mainstream prison population. Western Australia also has a policy of segregating those known to be antibody positive, but then it is difficult to see that this can do much good if the antibody status of the majority of prisoners remains unknown.

Another proposal advanced by the working party from the National Advisory Committee on AIDS (NACAIDS), and one receiving consideration in all states, is compulsory urine testing to determine whether prisoners are using intravenous drugs. The committee's suggestion is that those found to be using intravenous drugs be denied contact visits (that is, visits where there is body contact with the visitor) since these visits make it easy to transfer drugs to a prisoner.

In dealing with the problem of AIDS within the prison situation there seem to be two basic strategies. The first, the NACAIDS strategy, is to supply condoms and make renewed efforts to keep out intravenous drugs. The second, the South Australian strategy, is to have compulsory antibody testing and segregation of antibody positive prisoners from antibody negative ones. The latter strategy involves making further inroads upon the civil liberties of the prisoner. The former makes the assumption that it is possible to accomplish what has to date proved impossible, namely a drug-free prison.

ADDITIONAL READING

Duckett, M. *Australia's Response To AIDS* Canberra: Australian Government Publishing Service, 1986

Hancock, G. and Carim, E. *AIDS: The Deadly Epidemic* London: Gollancz, 1986

Nelkin, D. and Hilgartner, S. 'Disputed Dimensions of Risk: A Public School Controversy over AIDS' *The Milbank Quarterly* 64, Supplement 1, 1986

NSW Mental Health Act, 1983, No. 178. 5(1) (a); 5(1) (b)

QUESTIONS

1 How would you feel about a classmate if you knew he/she was infected with the AIDS virus ?
2 Should a student infected with the AIDS virus be able to attend school? Does his/her age make a difference?
3 Should the teacher be informed if a child is HIV antibody positive? Does the age of the child make a difference?
4 Do the parents of other children in the school have a right to know if a child in the school is HIV antibody positive?

10 THE PROVISION OF HEALTH CARE

NANCY: Did anyone hear that news about AIDS this morning?

BILL: You mean the stuff about Africa and how they think some huge percentage of the population already have the disease?

CHRISTINE: How are they going to explain to primitive people how not to get AIDS, how they must use condoms and all that? And even if they could stop more people getting the virus, how can a poor country afford to pay the costs of those who already have it?

NANCY: That's not just a problem in Africa, you know. In the United States some health insurance companies do not want to cover people who are infected with the AIDS virus.

CHRISTINE: So what happens to them?

NANCY: Well, in some states it has been made illegal to exclude people who are antibody positive.

BILL: That seems unreasonable to me. After all, people with other serious diseases can be excluded by health insurance companies, so why not those who are antibody positive? If you smoke or are overweight you have to pay higher premiums. But that's only fair: if you choose to take risks you should have to pay for the consequences.

CHRISTINE: We're lucky to have Medicare. At least it ensures that everyone is covered for treatment in public hospitals.

BILL: But then we all have to pay for that treatment through our taxes, and medical care is very expensive. The fact that we have to pay for all those smokers means that there is less money to fund student places in universities.

CHRISTINE: But Bill, there are lots of diseases and disabilities that people are not responsible for. Take multiple sclerosis. Nobody knows why some people get it. It's just a matter of being lucky or unlucky. If someone is unlucky enough to have that, why should he be further penalised by having to pay the full costs of his expensive medical treatments?

NANCY: That's right. After all, Bill, it's just luck that you or I don't have MS — or something just as bad.

BILL: Well, I agree that in the case of multiple sclerosis we should help the person pay his medical costs. But what about people who smoke and then get lung cancer? That case seems very different to me. And AIDS too. Everyone knows that you get AIDS from dirty needles and unsafe sex. If someone chooses to take those risks that's fine by me — so long as I'm not expected to pay for his health care when he gets sick.

CHRISTINE: But AIDS and lung cancer are very different. The people who have AIDS now didn't know they were putting themselves at risk when they shared needles and had unsafe sex. Most of those who now have AIDS probably caught it before there was any information.

BILL: But what about those who are engaging in risky practices now, after all the publicity there has been? Should we have to pay for their medical treatments when they go into hospital three or five years from now? I can't see any reason why we should.

NANCY: Your position is fine in theory, Bill, but it's just not practical. In three or five or ten years there are still going to be people who get AIDS through no fault of their own. What are you going to do about the wife who doesn't know her husband is bisexual? She gets AIDS. It's not her fault he lied to her, so why should she be further punished by having to pay her own medical costs?

BILL: She shouldn't be. The person should only pay if it's her fault that she has the disease.

NANCY: But to find out whether the person was at fault you'd have to have their private life investigated in tremendous detail. It simply is not acceptable to invade the privacy of individuals in that way and it would cost so much you might just as well pay for the medical treatment of everyone who needs it.

BILL: Maybe there are some difficult cases, but there are easy ones too. Doctors can tell if someone is an intravenous drug user.

CHRISTINE: The intravenous drug user is probably addicted, and not in any position to be able to give up drugs. Society makes it worse by making it difficult to have access to clean needles. I don't think you can hold an addict responsible for getting AIDS.

BILL: Okay, forget about AIDS for the moment. What about heavy smokers who get lung cancer? Why the hell should we pay for their medical costs?

NANCY: Maybe in theory we shouldn't. But what else can we do? We're not going to leave them to die on the streets, are we?

There are many things that individuals need and for which the average person then pays the market price. Take a house or apartment. In the majority of cases an individual will decide whether he or she wants two or three bedrooms, harbour views, and a swimming pool. The individual will be constrained in making his or her decision by the amount he or she is able to spend. How much one is prepared to sacrifice is also relevant. For example, would the purchaser be prepared to go without holidays, sell the car or get a second job? With respect to the purchase of a house the individual usually pays the full price. If one cannot afford to buy the sort of house one would like, then one must settle for something less. If one cannot afford any kind of house then one cannot become a home owner.

One method for delivering medical care is to have a market in medical care similar to our present market in real estate. With this system — call it system A — each individual will pay the full costs of his or her health care, and if the individual cannot afford to pay then he or she will go without.

System A has one very real advantage — it is a system that makes no claim on the public purse. But most of us have some misgivings about this system. Take the case of baby Kim who was born with a hole in the heart. If she does not undergo a sophisticated operation then she is almost certain to die before she reaches school age. And take Bill. Until he reached the age of twelve Bill was perfectly normal, but then tragically it was discovered that Bill was developing a curvature of the spine. Again medical science can do something for Bill. He can be put in traction for long periods of time so that his spine is mechanically straightened. It's reasonably effective, but very expensive.

There are also those who are unlucky enough to be involved in serious accidents. Amy is one of these: the car in which she was travelling collided with a semi-trailer carrying a load of gasoline. Amy was badly burned in the conflagration which followed, but the doctors managed to save her life. Now in order that she have some chance of leading something like a normal life it is necessary for her to have extensive plastic surgery to repair the damage inflicted by her burns.

Individuals born with serious medical problems, those born with a propensity to develop such conditions later in life, and those unfortunate enough to be involved in serious accidents are all at a disadvantage with respect to the average healthy individual. It seems unfair that those who are disadvantaged in this way should also have to bear the full financial costs of paying for treatments for their problems.

It is thinking of this kind that has motivated many to argue for publicly funded health insurance for all members of the community. Under such an arangement an individual's access to medical care will not be limited by his or her ability to pay. Baby Kim can have her heart operation, Bill his traction and Amy her plastic surgery even if their parents are penniless.

Public funding of medical care may take many forms. Let's start with a very straightforward system which we will call system B. Under system B an individual consults a doctor whenever he or she needs to, and is then able to obtain a refund from the government for the full cost of his or her treatment. Similarly, if one has to go into hospital for more lengthy or complicated treatments one is able to recover any expenditures one makes.

While accomplishing the laudable aim of providing more equitable access to medical care, a system like system B, where the government pays all the costs of an individual's medical treatments, is likely to be very expensive. More specifically, it will be open to abuse when patients overutilise services because they are 'free'. Mary doesn't feel very well. It's nothing serious, but since she hasn't anything better to do, and because it's free, she goes to see her doctor. But while it may be 'free' to Mary, her trip to the doctor does have to be paid for — by the taxpayer.

Patients are not the only ones able to abuse such a system. Medical practitioners may overservice patients at an enormous cost to the taxpayer. Mary goes to the doctor because she has an infection. The doctor takes a swab. He sends it to the pathologist, who is a member of the same practice, and requests twenty tests. It's highly unlikely that all these tests are really necessary, but why not have them? It's to the doctor's advantage to order them since the pathologist is a member of his own practice. If it costs Mary nothing, she will have no reason to prevent the doctor from requesting them. Indeed since there is some slight chance that the infection is caused by an unusual organism it's in her interests to have all twenty.

No country in the world uses system B in the pure form in which I have sketched it. One way or another system B has been modified to control the costs of running it. In Britain most general practitioners are salaried workers who are paid according to the number of patients on their books rather than according to the number of consultations they have (and there is a limit to the number of patients any one doctor may have). This system effectively eliminates overservicing instigated by the medical practitioner, but it will not completely remove the problem of patient-initiated overservicing for patient demand may still result in the employment of doctors additional to the number that are strictly necessary.

The other major problem with the British National Health System is that it reduces patient choice. Each doctor is limited to a given number of patients, and this means that patients frequently will not have access to the doctor of their choice. Furthermore, doctors have little incentive to improve the quality or efficiency of their service since this cannot result in their earning higher incomes.

Australia differs from Britain in that most Australian doctors are paid by Medicare on the basis of the number of consultations they have. Medicare is funded by a 1.25 per cent levy on income tax which everyone must pay regardless of the amount of medical care he or she needs. Thus, the rich and healthy subsidise the health care costs of the poor and ill. However Medicare is not without its problems. It is proving to be far more expensive to run than was originally anticipated. In the first place there is the problem of overservicing. In the second there are the costs associated with running the massive Medicare bureaucracy.

Australia has attempted to contain the problem of overservicing by requiring the individual to pay for a percentage — usually 15 per cent — of the cost of the treatments received. However, since the higher income earner is already paying a large and compulsory Medicare levy there still exists an incentive for that person to 'get his or her money's worth'. The 15 per cent deductible will be insufficient to dissuade the more affluent from consuming medical care. It will only prove effective in the case of those least able to pay. Increasing the size of the deductible will cut down on waste, and simultaneously make the system more inequitable as an increasing number of lower income earners cannot afford to pay the deductible.

Is there a system of funding medical care which is both equitable and non-wasteful? Maybe there is no system that is simultaneously perfect in both respects but there may still be some that are better than others.

One way of organising our thoughts on this matter is to use a device constructed by John Rawls. In his book *A Theory of Justice*, Rawls suggests that a system of ethical principles is fair or just, if it is the one we would choose from behind a 'veil of ignorance'. Imagine that we inhabit some pre-natal world. We know nothing about ourselves — neither how rich, nor intelligent, nor healthy we will be after birth. Rawls suggests that the ethical principles we would choose under these circumstances are likely to take account of the concerns of persons from all walks of life, and will not favour special interest groups since when we are behind the veil of ignorance we do not know which interest groups we will belong to after we are born.

The Rawlsian approach is useful because it helps us divorce ourselves from our immediate concerns and interests, and tries to develop ethical rules we would choose were we not blinded by day-to-day demands and our own particular advantages. More specifically it provides a very useful device for helping us to apportion (scarce) resources.

Medical care costs money, but then so do schools, universities, highways and airports. A nation has a large, but finite, amount of money to spend on the provision of public services. If we had unlimited resources governments would have fewer problems, but in the real world resources are always limited.

So what kinds of misfortune would individuals behind the veil of ignorance choose to insure themselves against? It seems plausible to argue that such individuals would favour a system of medical insurance in which they are at least protected should they be born with chronically bad health, or suffer some catastrophic injury since these individuals are the very ones who will find it impossible to obtain reasonable cost insurance through the private market. If a person is born with haemophilia it will be impossible for him or her *at that point* to obtain low cost insurance since insurance companies will know that there is a high probability the person will require costly medical treatment. In contrast, if a person is born with the predisposition to develop a serious illness which only shows up later in life, he or she will be able to obtain low cost medical insurance against that contingency early on in life, since the insurance company will have no more reason than the individual has to suspect that that person is a bad risk.

It is not simply bloody mindedness that causes private health insurance companies to act the way they do. Like any business, a health insurance company expects to make a profit, and like any business it passes on its costs of operation to its customers. Suppose now that governments forced insurance companies to offer health insurance at the same price to all individuals whether or not those individuals had serious diseases. What would happen in such a situation is that the insurance premiums of all customers would rise to an extent that would allow the company to pay for the costs of treatments required by those individuals with serious diseases. The cost of health insurance premiums can only be kept down if insurance companies can eliminate those with very costly illnesses from their clientele. It is in the interests of the 'healthy' purchaser of insurance to keep unhealthy individuals out of his or her scheme because only then will he or she be able to purchase reasonably priced health insurance on the private market.

But what of those unhealthy individuals who have had the misfortune to be born with, or to have accidently acquired, serious medical conditions? Where there is information available to the insurance company that an individual has, or is likely to have, such an illness that individual will not be able to purchase moderate cost health insurance through the private market. Individuals choosing from behind the veil of ignorance would be most likely to vote for this kind of insurance. Thus, a system of post-natal redistribution of medical resources which duplicates the missing pre-natal medical insurance can be provided with an ethical justification using the Rawlsian strategy.

A POSSIBLE OBJECTION

Does the Rawlsian justification for the redistribution of medical resources open a Pandora's box so that many other forms of redistribution may be justified on the same grounds?

When we are behind the veil of ignorance, as mentioned earlier, we do not know whether we will be rich or poor, intelligent or stupid, healthy or unhealthy. Now since a chance exists that I will be born into a poor family would it not then be rational for me (and all other individuals behind the veil) to contract for an insurance policy which redistributes income to me on the off-chance that I am born poor?

Let's look at an example. Suppose the government collected everything which was produced in a society, and redistributed it equally among all its members. In such a society an individual would have little incentive to push himself or herself to maximise his or her production since the amount each individual receives is essentially independent of the amount he or she contributes. In such a society many individuals would attempt to 'free ride' off the work of other members, and the result would be that the amount of goods available for redistribution was greatly diminished. This problem — a problem which economists refer to as the problem of *moral hazard* — would raise the costs of providing such insurance so much that no one behind the veil of ignorance would want to purchase it.

A less extreme case is one in which the government collects sufficient from the more affluent members of the society to pay for certain basic necessities for the least well off members of the society. Again such an arrangement could be expected to result in some free riding. More specifically, some of those individuals who were badly off though not sufficiently impoverished to qualify for government assistance would decide to reduce their efforts to provide for themselves and simply accept what is offered to them by the government.

Would individuals behind the veil of ignorance want to provide themselves with such insurance? Presumably so. What is of interest here, however, is how much free riding is tolerable before the cost of 'income insurance' becomes so high that no one behind the veil of ignorance would wish to purchase it. This issue is one that is now receiving a great deal of attention worldwide for it is simply the old and familiar question: how much social welfare should a nation provide for its citizens?

But the redistribution of medical resources is less plagued with problems of moral hazard than the redistribution of income. In the first place, nothing can be done by an individual to alter his or her endowed health status. Secondly, nothing can be done by an individual to avert an unforeseeable medical catastrophe. Finally, there are natural barriers to the consumption of medical care. Most people have some aversion to being ill, so the provision of medical insurance will not lead them to neglect their health completely, since that has other costs — like feeling terrible — that the individual alone will bear.

Some redistribution of medical resources seems both economically feasible and ethically justified. However, this still leaves open the question of what form this redistribution is to take. As noted earlier, a system of redistribution of medical resources such that all medical expenses are paid by the taxpayer — system B — will be open to abuse from both patients and doctors, and this will result in waste.

The British have attempted to curtail medical care expenditures with their system of salaried doctors. Australia has sought to achieve the same end by requiring the individual to pay a percentage of his or her medical bills over and above the Medicare tax levy which he or she cannot avoid paying. Australian medical care expenditure could be further curtailed if Australian doctors were forced to become salaried employees of the state, but for various historical and sociological reasons this is not a suggestion to which they could be expected to respond enthusiastically.

There are other reasons for seeing doctors as salaried employees as a less than optimal solution. If we set the prices for medical services artificially low, doctors currently practising medicine will make less money than they do now, but all this may do is encourage them to migrate to other countries, change professions or to provide a lower quality of service. In addition, if the supply of medical services falls too dramatically, the available supply will be rationed by consumers queueing for services. The costs of waiting in doctors' surgeries and for operations will be born by those patients seeking medical treatment, and these costs will not be counterbalanced by gains to anyone, which is of course an inefficient utilisation of resources.

The kinds of arguments outlined above are often advanced by those opposed to any move toward nationalised health care services. However, in the interests of accuracy it should be noted that even without Medicare the Australian health care system would be a far cry from a genuine market operation. In the first place entry to the profession is in the hands of the profession itself. This is particularly notable in the medical specialities — anaesthetics, surgery, radiology etc — where the college in question decides how many new members it will admit. Undoubtedly this accomplishes some desirable ends but it also acts as a device for ensuring that those already practicing in a particular speciality continue to enjoy high incomes. The second important point to note is that medical 'professional ethics' disallow any possibility of genuine market competition. For example, individual doctors are not allowed to advertise 'cut-price' services or criticise their colleagues' treatments.

Subsidised catastrophe insurance is one possible solution to the medical insurance problem. This is a system in which the state subsidises the health insurance premiums of individuals who are born with or accidentally acquire conditions which make their health much worse than the average person's. These people are part of the 'high-risk' group of individuals seeking insurance who would not be able to obtain insurance in a free competitive market at the rate available to 'low-risk' individuals. In this system non-catastrophic medical expenses would be borne by the individual, who would either pay for them out of his or her own pocket or through medical insurance from the private market.

Such a scheme would reduce the national Medicare bill. However it would do nothing for those low income individuals who cannot afford to pay for even their non-catastrophic medical treatments. Furthermore, what begins as a non-catastrophe may well develop into one if left untreated. Take three-year-old Sue who falls and cuts her leg. Sue's parents are too poor to take her to the doctor, and because she has not had an injection she develops tetanus. It's not Sue's fault that she cut her leg — it was an accident. And its not her fault either that her parents are too poor to pay for any medical treatment. She is just unlucky.

Considerations of equity will again push us in the direction of a health care scheme under which very low income individuals will have their non-catastrophic medical insurance premiums paid for, or at least subsidised by the government. The fine tuning of this kind of scheme may again require the consumer to pay for a portion of the costs of his or her treatments to discourage over-utilisation of services.

THE AIDS BILL

According to recent estimates, the medical care costs of people with AIDS in the United States in 1985 came to US$630 million. In comparison, in 1985 in the United States US$5.6 billion was spent on the health care of road accident victims, US$3.4 billion on those suffering from cancer of the respiratory tract, and US$2.2 billion on women suffering from breast cancer.

As yet health care expenditures on AIDS sufferers are comparatively low. What is disturbing is that the Center for Disease Control in Atlanta estimates that by 1991 the incidence of AIDS per 100 000 population will be 68.63 cases, as opposed to 3.96 cases per 100 000 population in 1984. This will put medical care expenditures on AIDS second only to those on road accident victims.

Australia can expect to see a similar escalation in the number of cases of AIDS in the years to come. At the end of December 1987 Australia had had 681 cases of AIDS. It is estimated that there will be 1200 cases by the end of 1988, and 3000 cases by December 1990.

The popular press has made much of the distinction between innocent and non-innocent victims of AIDS. The innocent are those who did not acquire HIV through homosexual sex or intravenous drug use. Children, haemophiliacs, and the spouses of covert intravenous drug users or bisexuals are the paradigmatic innocents.

But this innocent/non-innocent distinction with respect to HIV infection is not well-founded. To date probably the majority of the so-called non-innocent have acquired HIV in *total innocence* of the fact that the activities they were involved in carried with them the danger of infection. Until very recently it was not known that intravenous drug use and homosexual sex could result in the transmission of HIV.

Whatever else one may argue, it is not reasonable to argue that individuals who acquired HIV through intravenous drug use or homosexual sex had some privileged access to the fact that they were putting themselves at risk. They had no more knowledge that they were doing this than the recipient of a transfusion or a monogamous spouse.

Another point is that even when individuals are infected as a result of activities they know to be dangerous, it is rather inappropriate to label them guilty. Foolish or stupid may be appropriate descriptions. But guilty? Do we label lung cancer victims guilty if they have gone on smoking despite the well-publicised evidence of a connection between smoking and lung cancer?

Some may argue that there is a basis for treating individuals with self-inflicted injuries or illnesses differently from those whose injuries and illnesses are not self-inflicted. The paradigmatic example of a self-inflicted disease is lung cancer in a heavy smoker. It is now well established, and also well publicised, that cigarette smoking causes lung-cancer. So, it may be argued, if an individual decides to smoke why should the community pay his or her medical bills when he or she is hospitalised with lung cancer?

If it could be easily and cheaply ascertained which individuals were suffering from self-inflicted illnesses and injuries then there would be a strong case for not providing them with subsidised health care. The problem, however, is that it is not easy to ascertain these things. The first difficulty is that the kind of investigation needed to determine whether an individual is suffering from a self-inflicted illness will often involve unacceptable substantive intrusions into his or her privacy. The second objection is that establishing that the illness was self-inflicted could well cost the community as much as paying for the medical treatment.

A third objection has to do with the fact that in many cases of illness there is a genetic factor involved. Take Fred. He eats red meat three times a day. He also chain smokes and drinks heavily, but fortunate Fred comes from a line of strong genetic stock, and lives to the ripe old age of ninety with no medical problems — he dies when he is hit by a bus! Bruce, on the other hand, keeps to a low cholesterol diet and neither drinks nor smokes, but has had his first heart attack by forty. Bruce comes from a family with a predisposition toward heart attack — he is just unlucky. Now Barry. Barry also come from a family with a history of heart attack. He is a non-smoker. However, he does have the occasional meal of red meat and usually has a glass of wine with dinner. Barry makes it to 50 without a heart attack, but then he too is struck down.

Should the community pay for Bruce's medical care but not Barry's? This is not an easy question to answer. Barry has certainly shown some restraint with respect to his eating and drinking habits, though not as much as has Bruce. So what should we do? How should we decide? Any system of subsidised health care that differentiated between illnesses and injuries that are self-inflicted and those which are not would have to make judgements about cases like these and others even more difficult to decide upon.

Those individuals who now have AIDS or ARC fall within the class of individuals whose medical insurance/health care should be subsidised by the state since AIDS and ARC are conditions which, from behind the veil of ignorance, all individuals would agree to setting up institutions to provide insurance against. They are catastrophic misfortunes that no one could reasonably have been expected to foresee. Remember that until very recently no one knew that one could become infected with HIV through sexual intercourse or through sharing needles.

The health care of AIDS and ARC sufferers should continue to be subsidised by the state. There is of course the possibility that some who contract AIDS or ARC in the future will do so because they have *chosen* to engage in high-risk behaviour. However, given the obvious enormity of the problem of separating these individuals from the rest, and the fact that the latest scientific evidence indicates that there is a genetic component involved in determining susceptibility to the disease, the pragmatic solution is to subsidise the health care of all those who develop AIDS or ARC.

ADDITIONAL READING

Brown, M. C. *National Health Insurance in Canada and Australia* Canberra: The Health Economics Research Unit, Australian National University, 1985

OECD Social Policy Studies No. 4 *Financing and Delivering Health Care* Paris: OECD, 1987

Rawls, J. *A Theory of Justice* Oxford: Oxford University Press, 1972

QUESTIONS

1 What kinds of things do you think
   (a) individuals should pay for themselves?
   (b) the state should provide?
2 Suppose you won $50 000 dollars. How would you spend it?

3 Form a group — the bigger the better — and try, as a group, to answer question 2.
4 If you were Prime Minister how would you spend the money collected in taxation? Give a list of priorities but remember you only have a finite amount of money.
5 Form a group — the bigger the better — and try, as a group, to answer question 4.
6 Should people with AIDS be given financial assistance by the government to pay for their medical expenses? What about people with multiple sclerosis, heart disease, lung cancer? If you said yes in every case, try to formulate a general principle that covers all these cases as well as any others you would wish to include. If you said no in every case explain why. If you said yes sometimes and no sometimes, try to give a general reason why you included some cases but excluded others.

11 AIDS AND YOU

Much of this book has been concerned with looking at moral questions connected with the phenomenon of AIDS; questions like: How should individuals infected with HIV behave with respect to their sexual partners? How should society deal with HIV infected individuals who behave irresponsibly and thereby expose others to the risk of infection? Should the existence of AIDS cause us to modify our laws concerning intravenous drugs?

If we lived in a world in which everyone behaved in a morally responsible manner all the time then we could expect that the incidence of AIDS, in the advanced western nations at least, would soon begin to fall. Unfortunately, however, we do not live in such a world. Individuals cannot be relied upon to always act in a way that will minimise the risk of transmitting AIDS to previously uninfected individuals.

Take Sally and Bill. Bill is in love with Sally and wants to move in with her. Sally is keen on Bill too but she is cautious about making any kind of long term commitment. Until a year ago Sally was unhappily married to Fred and she is not keen to repeat that particular mistake. Sally believes the reason that her marriage to Fred failed was because Fred was too countercultural. He liked smoking marijuana but very little else. As a result of her experience Sally is violently opposed to drug use of any kind.

Until recently Bill has used intravenous drugs though now he is in love with Sally he has stopped. Bill does not tell Sally about his past drug use, even though he has shared needles with other drug users and so is at risk of being infected with HIV. Why doesn't he tell her? Well, Bill is no fool. He knows that Sally is ambivalent about moving in with him. If he tells her about his intravenous drug use this could make her decide against the move. It's not hard to see why people do not always do the morally right thing. Often it's just so much easier to do the wrong thing and hope that you will be lucky and nothing bad happen.

With respect to the transmission of HIV, particularly with respect to its sexual transmission, strong emotions are frequently involved. Take Nancy. She is in love with Jack. Her previous boyfriend, Nick, was bisexual but Nancy was not aware of this. Nancy only found out accidentally from a mutual friend. Needless to say she felt angry and humiliated. Nancy now needs a new relationship so that she can re-establish a feeling of self-worth. She does not tell Jack that her ex-boyfriend was bisexual — it's partly pride and partly fear that it may result in her losing Jack.

With something as serious as AIDS it is just not sensible to hope that other people will always do the right thing. It's like using a pedestrian crossing — better to look both ways before you step out even though the pedestrian does have right of way and vehicles are obliged by law to stop for anyone using a crossing. Failure to take the extra and simple precaution of looking before stepping out onto the crossing can have terrible consequences for an individual. It is small consolation to someone permanently confined to a wheelchair to know that the motorist was in the wrong.

AIDS leads to death, and it is not a pleasant death. The opportunistic infections associated with AIDS are serious and painful. Pneumocystis pneumonia leads to debilitation and dramatic weight loss. Karposi's sarcoma brings about disfiguring cancerous lesions of the skin. Cytomegalovirus attacks the lungs and eyes, and can lead to blindness. Cryptococcus causes severe meningitis and Candida albicans (or thrush) can occur so thickly in throat and mouth that swallowing becomes problematic. With AIDS the patient's body will be simultaneously ravaged by a number of these serious diseases.

Getting ARC is not pleasant either. There are swollen glands, diarrhoea, night sweats and high temperatures. It affects your work and your social life.

If one is fortunate enough to escape AIDS and ARC, the HIV virus can attack the brain directly. The result is a gradual dementia with its concomitant mood swings, loss of physical coordination and linguistic abilities. Once in the brain the AIDS virus can also be responsible for symptoms which mimic conditions as varied as schizophrenia and multiple sclerosis. One American expert, Dr Paul Volberding, head of AIDS services at San Francisco General

Hospital, has said, 'It is entirely reasonable to speculate that *everyone* who is seropositive will develop central nervous system complications.' (Hancock and Carim, 1986: 28)

Once one is infected with the HIV virus, AIDS, ARC and dementia become frighteningly real possibilities. According to the World Health Organisation the probability of developing AIDS within five years of infection is between 10 and 30 per cent, and the probability of developing ARC in that same five year period between 20 and 50 per cent. The probability of dementia or other neurological complications in the long run may well be 100 per cent.

SO HOW CAN I AVOID CATCHING AIDS?

The one good thing about the AIDS virus is that it's not like a cold or flu virus. You can't catch it just by being in the same room as someone who is infected with HIV. Apart from babies who catch it from their mothers, and individuals who get it as a result of a transfusion (which is now highly unlikely), the two most likely ways of catching HIV are through sharing needles or syringes, and through unprotected sex.

Needles and syringes

If someone infected with HIV uses a needle or syringe to inject himself or herself then small amounts of blood will be left on it. This blood may contain HIV. So if you use the syringe after an infected person has used it you can be injecting the HIV virus directly into your own bloodstream. The probability of infection if one uses an HIV contaminated needle is very high. If you are an intravenous drug user, it is very important that you follow these guidelines, in order to avoid the possibility of becoming infected with the HIV virus:

1. Don't use a dirty needle and that means *any* needle that someone else has used. It is irrelevant that it may look clean. The droplets of blood harbouring the HIV virus may be so tiny that they are invisible to the naked eye. So use clean needles, or your own needle that no one else has ever used.

2. If you have to use a needle that someone else has used then cover it with water and boil it for at least 10 minutes.
3. If you can't boil it then soak it in at least 20 per cent alcohol, (eg methylated spirits, gin or rum) for at least an hour. Remember, it must be totally submerged. Before using it again rinse it with water to get rid of the alcohol.
4. Finally, if you can't wait an hour then rinse the syringe at least five times before using it. It's better to use 20 per cent alcohol, but if you don't have that, water is still better than nothing. Take the needle off, fill the syringe with alcohol, put the needle on and eject the alcohol/water. If you use alcohol the final rinse should be with water.

Remember, these strategies are not all equally effective. It is always best to use new disposable syringes but if you can't do that then move down the list until you find something you can do. Rinsing with water five times is better than doing nothing but it's not as safe as using a new syringe.

Sex

There is no way of telling whether a person is infected with HIV just by looking at him or her. A person can be infected with HIV and be infectious to others, but feel and look perfectly well. If the person is infected then the HIV virus will be present in blood, semen and vaginal fluids, and may be passed on in all these fluids. If you have sex with someone infected with HIV and this involves an exchange of body fluids then you are at risk of becoming infected.

There are a number of ways of reducing the risk of catching HIV through sex. The first and most effective way to protect oneself from becoming infected is not to have sex with anyone, for clearly if you don't have sex with anyone, then there is no risk that you will catch HIV that way!

Another way to cut down the risk of sexual transmission of the virus is monogamy — that is, having sex with only one person. However, monogamy in itself is no insurance against becoming infected with the virus since you are only safe if your partner is not infected. You can get AIDS while being totally faithful to someone, if that someone happens to be infected with HIV. The fact that he or she is being faithful to you now is irrelevant if he or she has been infected with HIV by some previous lover.

While monogamy cannot ensure that you will not become infected, promiscuity will increase the chance that you may be exposed to HIV. Each time you have sex with a person who is at risk of being infected with HIV you too expose yourself to the risk of infection. If you have sex with a lot of people it's unlikely that you will know them well, and so you will have little idea about whether or not they have been in the kinds of situations which could lead to their being HIV infected.

Something else to keep in mind is that if your partner (even your monogamous partner) has ever injected intravenous drugs with a dirty needle he or she is also at risk of being infected. That means you too may be at risk. Even if your partner is now off drugs, he or she may still have become infected on some previous occasion and that means you are now at risk.

Remember, it is possible to become infected with HIV by using *one dirty needle* or *having sex once* with an infected individual.

SAFE SEX

Another way to reduce the risk of catching HIV is to always use condoms in situations where there is an exchange of body fluids. This means using a condom *every time* one has vaginal or anal sex. It means putting the condom on correctly, and ensuring that there is no leakage from the condom after ejaculation. It means using a condom whenever there is penetrative sex and not just putting it on before orgasm. Remember, women have become pregnant because of sperm that has left the penis before the man ejaculates. If this fluid can result in pregnancy, it can also bring about AIDS.

How safe am I if I use a condom?

The answer to this question is that you are much safer than if you didn't but still not 100 per cent so. Remember that accidents are possible even if unlikely. If some of the fluid escapes from the condom and that fluid contains HIV then there is risk of infection.

Every year thousands of people are killed and seriously injured in car accidents. The fear of death and injury on the road may lead some individuals to give up going on vacation by car over long weekends. Others may decide that they will never go on long car trips but will fly or go by train instead. Maybe some (presumably very few) decide never to travel in any kind of motor vehicle. Most of us, however, do not go so far as to abandon motor transport entirely. Rather we make more minor adjustments that will lower the risk of our being killed or seriously injured on the roads — we always use seatbelts, we do not drive if we have been drinking, we do not drive long distances at night, but most of us will go on driving and travelling in cars at least some of the time.

Similarly we can expect that despite the threat of infection with HIV most individuals will choose to go on having sex at least some of the time. Each individual has to decide for himself or herself what is a reasonable level of risk. An individual is free to choose never to travel in a car if that individual wishes to minimise the risk that he or she will be killed or injured in a motor accident. Similarly an individual is free to decide never to have sex if he or she wishes to minimise the risk of becoming infected with HIV through sex. It's up to you to decide what is an acceptable level of risk for you. After all it's your body, and you are the one who will suffer if you get AIDS.

Not all sexual activities carry with them the same risks of infection with HIV. Activities like masturbation are generally very low risk. The following is a list of sexual behaviours and the relative risks of HIV infection associated with them. Some activities are low risk, some are high risk. Some are virtually risk free.

1 Sex, also known as fucking, screwing, etc. This usually means vaginal intercourse where the male inserts his penis into the female's vagina. The risk of HIV transmission is high for the female, moderate for the male.

2 Kissing. Ordinary social kissing — the proverbial 'peck on the cheek' — is without risk. 'French', 'tongue', or 'deep' kissing carries an unknown but presumably very low risk of transmission unless

AIDS AND YOU

either partner has cuts or ulcers in the mouth. In the latter case the risk is higher but still is presumably quite low.

3 Masturbation (male), otherwise known as jerking off, pulling yourself, wanking, whacking off, tossing off, etc., is where a male or female partner uses his or her hand to stimulate his or her partner's penis. Providing any skin that comes in contact with the semen is intact there is no risk.

4 Masturbation (female). This is where a male or female partner uses his or her hand to stimulate a partner's clitoris and genital area. Again, so long as any skin that comes into contact with vaginal secretions is intact, there is no risk.

5 Fellatio, also known as going down on, giving head, sucking off, or a blow job. This is where a male or female partner uses his or her mouth to stimulate a male partner's penis. The risk for the receptive partner is moderate to high depending on that partner's state of oral hygiene and whether or not the ejaculate is swallowed. The risk for the insertive partner is unknown but presumed to be low.

6 Cunnilingus, also known as going down on, eating, licking out. This is where a male or female partner uses his or her mouth to stimulate a female partner's genital area. The risks for both partners are unknown but presumed to be low.

7 Anal intercourse, also known as fucking, Greek fucking, buggering, etc. This is where a male partner inserts his penis into a male or female partner's anus. If a condom is not used the risk is extremely high for the receptive partner, and moderate to high for the insertive partner. If a condom is used the risks for both partners are lower. However, there is still some risk for the condom may tear or there may be spillage of ejaculate from the condom.

8 Sadomasochism, otherwise known as S & M. This is where one partner inflicts pain upon the other as an aid to sexual arousal. Sadomasochistic practices are safe so long as there is no exchange of body fluids.

The activities listed above carry with them different risks of infection with the HIV virus. While in many cases the risk involved has not been studied in sufficient detail to give it an exact numerical value it is still possible, given what is known about the nature of HIV and its mode of transmission, to make a rough assessment of that risk. The picture which emerges is one in which some of the more ordinary sexual activities carry with them significant, and sometimes very high, risks. Unprotected vaginal intercourse with a male infected with HIV is a risky activity for his female partner. If the partners engage in anal rather than vaginal intercourse then the risk for the female becomes even higher.

For those who are concerned to at least reduce the risk of becoming infected with HIV the message here is very clear. Using a condom will significantly lower the risk, and will have other important advantages too. Using a condom lowers the risk of becoming pregnant (that's why condoms were invented) and it also lowers (though it does not totally eliminate) the risk of catching a number of other sexually transmitted diseases.

In most western societies including Australia sexually transmitted diseases (STDs) occur predominantly in the 15-30-year-old age group. Studies also show that the most common source of infection is a 'casual' sexual partner. Some sexually transmitted diseases, if left untreated, can be very serious. Gonorrhoea is a highly contagious STD which is spread primarily through sexual intercourse. In women symptoms can be non-existent or so slight that they are not noticed. However, the infection can destroy the fallopian tubes, and cause pelvic inflammatory disease which may lead to sterility. If an infected woman becomes pregnant the foetus may become infected with the gonococcal organism and this can cause blindness in the child.

Syphilis is another serious STD but one which, fortunately, does have symptoms in both sexes. Between nine and ninety days after infection the person develops a hard painless chancre (ulcer) at the site of infection. Two to four months later the infected person experiences some one or more of a cluster of mild symptoms which may include fever, headaches and a rash which occurs in warm and moist sites such as the genital and anal areas, under the breasts and in the armpits. If left untreated an individual may develop tertiary lesions many years later. This can lead to severe conditions such as dementia, personality changes, deafness and blindness. It can also lead to death. If a woman with syphilis becomes pregnant and remains untreated, the foetus may be miscarried or the child may be stilborn. If the child is born alive it may suffer from facial abnormalities, blindness, deafness, dementia and personality disorders.

Genital herpes caused by the herpes simplex virus is now the most common STD in western countries. Medically it is not as serious a condition as either gonorrhoea or syphilis, but genital herpes is a significant problem because it can be very painful (particularly for women), there is no cure for it, and it can have unpleasant psychological effects on sexual relationships. Herpes first appears in the form of small blisters which after two to three days break down and erode away to form small shallow ulcers. At times, and particularly in women, the infected areas are extensive. They are also very painful. If the woman becomes pregnant there is some risk that the virus will be passed on to the foetus with serious consequences. The greatest risk is if the mother is suffering an attack at the time of delivery, but if the doctor is aware of this possibility, the child can be delivered by caesarean section.

Gonorrhoea, syphilis and genital herpes are just three of many sexually transmitted diseases. Because a condom provides a barrier between the sexual organs of the individuals engaged in intercourse it is able to provide some protection with respect to the transmission of STDs. Using condoms to lower the risk of becoming infected with HIV is therefore a strategy which also gives some protection against infection with other unpleasant diseases.

Using condoms will lower the risk of becoming infected with the HIV virus. But is there anything more that a person can do? For example, is there any way to ascertain whether a sexual partner is infected with HIV? Since you cannot tell by looking at a person whether or not he or she is infected with the HIV virus you are, for all practical purposes, reliant upon the honesty and moral character of your sexual partner with respect to this matter. Each person is himself or herself best able to ascertain the risk of being infected with HIV for that person, and usually only that person, will know the details of those events within his or her past life which may have resulted in the transmission of the virus.

In general, it is foolish to rely upon the honesty of a chance acquaintance. With respect to sexual activities that may lead to one's becoming infected with HIV it would be particularly foolish. Individuals typically feel few responsibilities toward strangers. They usually come to feel they have responsibilities toward others only as they develop longstanding relationships with them. Of course some people never come to develop these feelings of responsibility. History contains some famous cases of husbands who infected their wives with syphilis. For example, Karen Blixen, the author of *Out of Africa*, was given syphilis by her husband Bors. In general, it is true that individuals are more likely to behave responsibly toward others where there is a longstanding relationship. Statistical research done on the transmission of sexually transmitted diseases substantiates this fact. Most cases of infection with these diseases are the result of 'casual' sexual encounters.

If you have already decided in favour of a sexual encounter with a stranger, or near stranger, then it is better (from the point of view of your health, at least) to engage in mutual masturbation — an activity which is perfectly safe so long as no bodily fluids come in contact with cut or grazed skin — than to have sexual intercourse. If you must have intercourse it is better to use a condom than not to use one.

As in the case of intravenous drug use there are more and less effective means for protecting oneself from HIV infection. Having sex with no one is safer than always using condoms. But sex with condoms is safer than sex without. In the end, of course, it's up to you. You yourself must decide what risks you are prepared to take. But it's worth some serious thought for, after all, it's your body and you will be the one to bear the consequences.

ADDITIONAL READING

Brown, V. A. et al *Our Daily Fix* Sydney: Australian National University Press, 1986

Hancock, G. and Carim, E. *AIDS: The Deadly Epidemic* London: Gollancz, 1986

Llewellyn-Jones, D. *Herpes, AIDS and Other Sexually Transmitted Diseases* London: Faber, 1985

Llewellyn-Jones, D. *Every Woman* London: Faber, 1986

Llewllyn-Jones, D. *Every Man* Oxford: Oxford University Press, 1987

Mann, J. 'The Global Strategy for AIDS Prevention and Control' Geneva: World Health Organisation, May 5, 1987

Richardson, D. *Women and The AIDS Crisis* London: Pandora, 1987

QUESTIONS

1 How is the HIV virus transmitted from one person to another?
2 What are the most likely ways that an individual will become infected with the HIV virus?
3 Is it possible to tell whether someone is infected with HIV by looking at him or her?
4 If a person uses intravenous drugs what should he or she do to protect himself or herself from becoming infected with HIV?
5 What sexual activities put someone at high risk of becoming infected with the HIV virus? What activities put him or her at moderate risk?
6 If you have decided to have a sexual relationship with someone but are worried that you may be at risk of becoming HIV infected what precautions can you use to lower the risk?
7 'My boyfriend used to use intravenous drugs but not anymore, and we are in a monogamous relationship, so I can't be at risk of becoming infected with HIV.' Is the speaker as safe as she thinks? If not, why not?